NICE at 25

Marking its 25th anniversary, this fascinating collection examines the pioneering work of the National Institute for Health and Care Excellence (NICE).

Setting standards for the delivery of healthcare, issuing guidance on public health, and assessing and making recommendations on health technologies, NICE has attracted widespread international attention, emulation, and comment. The authors in this collection, drawn from a broad range of disciplinary backgrounds, offer analysis of key issues which have informed NICE's work, from the principles of health economics, to patient engagement, to the legal basis on which NICE operates.

Covering many of the most important themes within contemporary debates on health policy and management today, this insightful collection will interest students and researchers, as well as policy makers in the field.

Peter Littlejohns is Emeritus Professor of Public Health at King's College London, and the founding Clinical and Public Health Director of NICE. He has led on a number of international research programmes addressing ways of improving the effectiveness and efficiency of health services through fair prioritisation policies.

Keith Syrett is Professor of Health Law and Policy and Director of the Centre for Health, Law, and Society in the School of Law, University of Bristol, UK. He has written extensively on the legal regulation of resource allocation in healthcare, health technology assessment, and public health law.

NICE at 25

A quarter-century of evidence, values, and innovation in health

Edited by Peter Littlejohns and Keith Syrett

Routledge
Taylor & Francis Group

LONDON AND NEW YORK

First published 2025
by Routledge
4 Park Square, Milton Park, Abingdon, Oxon OX14 4RN

and by Routledge
605 Third Avenue, New York, NY 10158

Routledge is an imprint of the Taylor & Francis Group, an informa business

British Library Cataloguing-in-Publication Data
A catalogue record for this book is available from the British Library

Library of Congress Cataloging-in-Publication Data
Names: Littlejohns, Peter, editor. | Syrett, Keith, editor.
Title: NICE at 25 : a quarter-century of evidence, values, and innovation in health / edited by Keith Syrett and Peter Littlejohns.
Description: Abingdon, Oxon ; New York, NY : Routledge, 2024. | Includes bibliographical references and index.
Identifiers: LCCN 2024011081 (print) | LCCN 2024011082 (ebook) | ISBN 9781032817736 (paperback) | ISBN 9781032248936 (hardback) | ISBN 9781003501268 (ebook)
Subjects: LCSH: National Institute for Clinical Excellence (Great Britain) | Great Britain. National Health Service. | Medical care—Great Britain—Evaluation. | Medical care—Great Britain—Cost effectiveness. | Health services accessibility—Great Britian. | Medicine and state—Great Britain.
Classification: LCC RA395.G7 N53 2024 (print) | LCC RA395.G7 (ebook) | DDC 362.10941—dc23/eng/20240410
LC record available at https://lccn.loc.gov/2024011081
LC ebook record available at https://lccn.loc.gov/2024011082

ISBN: 978-1-032-24893-6 (hbk)
ISBN: 978-1-032-81773-6 (pbk)
ISBN: 978-1-003-50126-8 (ebk)

DOI: 10.4324/9781003501268

Typeset in Times New Roman
by Apex CoVantage, LLC

Contents

Figures

Tables

Contributors

Kalipso Chalkidou is Director of Health Financing and Economics at the World Health Organization and Visiting Professor at Imperial College London. Before that she was Head of Health Finance at The Global Fund to Fight AIDS, Tuberculosis and Malaria. Previously she was Professor and Director of Global Health Policy at Imperial College London. She is the founding director of NICE's international programme.

Victoria Charlton is a PhD student at the Department of Global Health and Social Medicine, King's College London, and a visiting lecturer at Imperial College London. Her professional background is in science policy. Victoria's research focuses on the role played by social and ethical values in NICE technology appraisal.

Kinanti Khansa Chavarina is a Project Associate at the Health Intervention and Technology Assessment Program (HITAP), under the Ministry of Public Health, Thailand. She works on supporting countries, such as Indonesia and the Philippines, on health technology assessment institutionalisation and other relevant programmes. She received her Master of Public Health Degree from the National University of Singapore.

Karl Claxton is a Professor of Health Economics in the Centre for Health Economics, University of York, UK. He was a founding member of the NICE Appraisal Committee in 1999 and served on various NICE Appraisal Committees until 2012. His research interests include methods for the economic evaluation of health technologies, Bayesian decision theory, innovation and pharmaceutical pricing policy.

Anthony J. Culyer is Emeritus Professor of Economics in the Department of Economics & Related Studies, and the Centre for Health Economics, at the University of York, UK. His main current research interests lie in deliberative methods of decision-making in health and health care policy and practice.

David J. Hunter is Emeritus Professor of Health Policy and Management, Population Health Sciences Institute, Newcastle University, UK; and Emeritus Professor, Global Policy Institute, School of Government and International Affairs, Durham University, UK. His research interests, spanning over 40 years, lie in health system transformation and public health; in policy formation and implementation; and in trade and health.

Michael P. Kelly is Professor and Senior Visiting Fellow in the Department of Public Health and Primary Care at the University of Cambridge. Between 2005 and 2014 he was the Director of the Centre for Public Health at NICE. From 2005 to 2007 he directed the methodology work stream for the World Health Organization's Commission on the Social Determinants of Health. His research interests include the philosophy of evidence-based medicine, health inequalities, and health related behaviour change.

Peter Littlejohns is Emeritus Professor of Public Health at King's College London, and the founding Clinical and Public Health Director of NICE. He has led on a number of international research programmes addressing ways of improving the effectiveness and efficiency of health services through fair prioritisation policies.

Fiona Pearce is a Senior Advisor to the Agency for Care Effectiveness (ACE), Singapore's national HTA agency, providing technical support to the Health Technology Assessment (HTA) and Consumer Engagement and Education (CEE) work streams. She is one of the founding members of ACE and was responsible for developing the HTA methods and processes which the agency uses to conduct evaluations of drugs and vaccines to inform national subsidy decisions.

Mark Sculpher is Professor of Health Economics and Director of the Centre for Health Economics, University of York, UK. His research interests relate to economic evaluation and health technology assessment, including applied research, methods development and policy analysis. He has been a member of the National Institute for Health and Care Excellence (NICE) Technology Appraisal Committee, the NICE Public Health Interventions Advisory Committee and NICE's Diagnostics Advisory Committee.

Ryan Jonathan Sitanggang is an International Cooperation Officer at the Health Intervention and Technology Assessment Program (HITAP), under the Ministry of Public Health, Thailand. He works on facilitating collaborations between HITAP and its partners through networks and platforms to strengthen the capacity for HTA research and promote the integration of HTA evidence into policy decisions. He received his Bachelor's degree in Community Public Health from Asia-Pacific International University in Thailand.

Sophie Staniszewska is Professor of Health Services Research at Warwick Medical School, University of Warwick, UK. Sophie's research focuses on developing the evidence base of patient and public involvement and engagement in research. She has worked with the NICE Public Involvement Programme for many years and currently sits on the NICE Implementation Strategy Group. With Sophie Werkö, Sophie was Co-chair of the Methods and Impact sub-group of the HTAi Patient and Citizen Involvement Interest Group.

Keith Syrett is Professor of Health Law and Policy and Director of the Centre for Health, Law, and Society in the School of Law, University of Bristol, UK. He has written extensively on the legal regulation of resource allocation in healthcare, health technology assessment, and public health law.

Yot Teerawattananon is the founder of the Thai Ministry of Public Health's Health Intervention and Technology Assessment Program (HITAP) and a visiting professor at Saw Swee Hock School of Public Health at the National University of Singapore. He is also a co-founder of the HTAsiaLink network and the International Decision Support Initiative (iDSI).

Albert Weale is Emeritus Professor of Political Theory and Public Policy, University College London. He is the author of a number of works on health policy as well as studies in modern social contract theory.

Sophie Söderholm Werkö is Director of International Relations at the Swedish Agency for Health Technology Assessment and Assessment of Social Services (SBU), Sweden. Her research interests encompass Patient and Public Involvement and Engagement in HTA and in Social Intervention Assessment (SIA). For many years she led the work on Patient Involvement at SBU and at the Swedish Council for Knowledge-Based Policy. With Sophie Staniszewska, Sophie was Co-Chair of the Methods and Impact sub-group of the HTAi Patient and Citizen Involvement Interest Group.

James Wilson is Professor of Philosophy at University College London. He has published widely on public health ethics, the philosophy of public policy, and on the ownership and governance of ideas and information. His research uses philosophy to help resolve practical problems, and uses practical problems to investigate gaps and weaknesses in existing philosophical theories. His book *Philosophy for Public Health and Public Policy: Beyond the Neglectful State* (Oxford University Press) was published in 2021.

Foreword

Ara Darzi

NICE was very nearly strangled at birth. Shortly after its launch as the National Institute for Clinical Excellence on 1 April 1999, the Government asked the new body to assess Glaxo Wellcome's anti-influenza drug Relenza (zanamavir), ahead of the winter flu season. The request provoked an angry response from Glaxo Wellcome, who were 'appalled' at the very idea that the drug might not be made available on the NHS and warned of 'potentially devastating consequences'. In the event NICE did not recommend Relenza and the prime minister, Tony Blair, held firm, refusing to overturn the decision.

It was the first of many such battles. NICE has never been far from controversy. But 25 years on it is still with us, and still fulfilling its core purpose – to provide authoritative guidelines on best practice and determine whether expensive new technologies in general, and pharmaceuticals in particular, are clinically and cost-effective and should be made available on the NHS.

It has not only survived but prospered. Today, it is recognised globally for its ground breaking work, and its guidelines and health technology assessments are downloaded internationally. Its influence is felt worldwide.

The issues with which it must wrestle are nevertheless as hard as ever. They involve unavoidable trade-offs that are often agonising and have provoked bitter clashes with both patient groups and pharmaceutical companies. It has been characterised as a 'death panel' and accused of 'condemning patients to an early grave'. To say no to a drug is a dreadful blow for the patients. Yet to say yes to a cost ineffective drug ultimately risks driving out the cost-effective.

As a minister myself in the Labour government from 2007–9, I advocated for patients to be guaranteed access to drugs and treatments approved by NICE in my NHS Review, *High Quality Care for All.* That right was later enshrined in the NHS Constitution. NICE has since continued to shape my thinking as a surgeon, research academic and innovator, and I am indebted to it, as are so many others.

The biggest threat to its existence came with the creation of the Cancer Drugs Fund in 2010, set up to pay for drugs deemed too expensive by NICE to be cost-effective. The fund rapidly exceeded its budget, was widely perceived as broken, and was reabsorbed into NICE in 2016.

Over time NICE's virtues have been recognised by all sides. Chief among them is that it shields ministers from decisions around cost-effectiveness and what the NHS should and should not provide that they are ill-equipped to take.

The publication of *NICE at 25* is therefore a moment for celebration. The book's opening chapter describes NICE's history while the remainder analyse the multiple perspectives – economic, political, scientific, ethical, philosophical, patient-centred and legal – that inform its work. The panel of distinguished authors assembled by its editors share a passion for NICE that makes the book an enthralling read.

The challenges ahead are as great as any in the past and the services provided by NICE never more needed. *NICE at 25* is an invaluable resource for clinician scientists, healthcare innovators, economists, policy professionals, patient advocates and all who prize the delivery of high-quality health care today and in the future.

Preface

After 13 unique years immersed in the early development of NICE and then a further ten years researching the principles of fair and equitable prioritisation of health care, which meant he became a critical friend of the Institute, Peter Littlejohns thought that his NICE days were over. He resolved that there would be no more thinking or writing about the organisation! He was finally implementing his own guidance – over the last two decades he had warned many clinicians, patients and academics when asked about getting involved with NICE – 'be careful it is a very addictive institution'. Then he received an email from Keith Syrett on 3rd February 2021 (in the spirit of openness and transparency it is presented complete below):

Dear Peter

Apologies for emailing you out of the blue, but I wanted to put a tentative proposal to you which might perhaps be of interest.

NICE's 25th birthday isn't too far away now, of course, and I thought it would be good to put together a volume to 'celebrate' this. My thought was that it could be an edited collection written from a social science perspective, with chapters representing various different relevant disciplines (just off the top of my head and certainly not exhaustive: law, economics, ethics, health policy/systems, political science, etc.). The chapters could offer some sort of retrospective reflection from those perspectives, or an exploration of a particular question or issue which is of interest, whether contemporary or historical.

I've sounded out a publisher – Routledge – on a very informal, preliminary level, and they have indicated that they would be interested. In principle the aim would be to publish the book in 2024, to coincide with the anniversary.

I wonder what you might think of this idea and most importantly at this early stage – whether you might perhaps consider taking a role as an editor, alongside me? It would look very good, I think, both to publishers and, in due course to purchasers, to have the 'imprint' of someone who was closely connected with the Institute on the book. I am sure that you are much better connected than me, too (though I do have a number of names in mind). And I would hope, with a careful choice of reliable contributors, that the editorial task would not prove especially onerous! But of course I shall fully understand if your other commitments don't allow.

How could he resist? All his previous promises to himself evaporated. The following three years flew by as an efficient and synergistic working partnership emerged. In true post-Covid style the editors never met and have had only two virtual conversations. We think that when you read the book that you will agree the relationship has been very productive.

Peter Littlejohns and Keith Syrett, December 2023

Acknowledgements

Peter Littlejohns would like to thank Keith Syrett for his invitation to be co-editor and postponing his retirement for three years. But he would not have had it any other way. It was a fitting final project.

Peter would also like to thank all his colleagues and friends who became chapter writers and his wife Tercia for her love and support during the preparation of the book and in all other aspects of his life. Most especially, for encouraging him 25 years ago to apply for the inaugural NICE Clinical Director post. And finally his children Sam and Anna whose approach to public service inspires him daily.

Keith Syrett would like to express his profound gratitude to his co-editor, Peter Littlejohns, for his willingness to embark upon this project. Without Peter's associations, this book would simply never have been possible. He thanks him also for his considerable patience, perceptive suggestions, and wise advice during the process of putting the book together.

Keith would also like to thank all of the chapter authors for their excellent contributions to this volume, and his family for their love and support.

Albert Weale thanks the members of the KCL/UCL Social Values Group for all their thoughts on these issues over the years.

James Wilson would like to thank the editors, and Victoria Charlton, for helpful comments on earlier drafts of this chapter.

Michael P. Kelly led the teams which worked on the application of evidence-based principles to public health at the Health Development Agency and then was the Director of the Centre for Public Health Excellence at NICE until 2014. There were many colleagues whose work over the years helped to shape the way that the story unfolded. The teams that worked in the HDA and NICE were of course, central, and did much of the graft which produced the methods and the guidelines. The members of PHIAC, and the other independent advisory committees were also critical in helping shape the thinking which went on inside the organisation. The Chief Executive and the Chair of NICE during most of the period covered by this chapter, Sir Andrew Dillon and Sir Mike Rawlins, were steadfast in their support of the public health programme. Beyond NICE and the HDA, of particular importance are Catherine Law, Jenny Griffin, Dame Sally Davies, Christine McGuire, Mike Hoorah, Don Nutbeam, Fiona Adshead, and Simon Reeves. As serving past and present officials, their particular contributions have to remain invisible, but their support and help, made a real difference, and facilitated bringing the vision in the original Department of Health Strategy of 2001 to reality.

Sophie Staniszewska and Sophie Söderholm Werkö wish to acknowledge NICE colleagues who were able to supply a timeline with key milestones and links to reports, some of which would have been difficult to identify as the website only contains current information. We thank Victoria Thomas and her team for this input, particularly Heidi Livingstone and Laura Norburn. Many of the key developments are not necessarily reported in documents and papers and we have relied on their collective knowledge to help us identify key steps and for this, we as the authors, are very grateful. Lastly, we would also like to express our gratitude to NICE for, perhaps unknowingly, taking on a leadership role in patient and public involvement in the international HTA sphere – many agencies in several countries globally have benefitted from these significant developments. While not a revolution, NICE has enabled a significant evolution of working in partnership with patients and the public.

1   Introduction

Why NICE and why the book?

Peter Littlejohns and Keith Syrett

On 1 April 1999 the National Institute for Clinical Excellence (known as NICE) was established. Over the last 25 years, whenever quality in the NHS is discussed or debated, opinions (both favourable or otherwise) on NICE are never far behind. The Institute has seen numerous quality-related NHS organisations come and go, but has gradually expanded its brief from clinical medicine to public health and social care. There are few areas in health and social care today where NICE guidance does not describe the quality of service provision that professionals aspire to, and that patients expect.

The quarter-century anniversary of its founding provides a fitting moment to take stock of how the Institute has performed, explore the reasons why it has been successful when so many other institutions have fallen by the wayside, and to consider how it should adapt to the challenges still facing the NHS 25 years on.

In this introductory chapter we will first describe the circumstances that led to its creation and the landmarks in its expansion. However, this book is not meant primarily to be a history of NICE; rather it takes as its starting point the most important principle underpinning NICE's methods – that its guidance should be based on the best available evidence. We explore the types of social science and evidence required to inform and explain the workings and the outputs of NICE. We have identified eight key perspectives – Health Economics, Political Science, Health Policy, Ethics, Philosophy, Public Health, Patient and Public Involvement, and Law. As described further below, there is a chapter for each of these, written by authors who have been closely associated with NICE, either participating in, or commenting upon, the functions and activities of NICE over its long history. We also explore the international impact of the Institute.

The Institute is established

After 18 years of a Conservative government, in May 1997 Tony Blair's New Labour government came to power with a massive majority (the largest of any party since 1931). Part of its electoral appeal was its promise to reassert the

DOI: 10.4324/9781003501268-1

founding principles of the NHS and provide consistent standards of care. The variation in care it had inherited was epitomised by the differing access across the country to expensive new drugs, especially those for cancer. The popular press characterised this as the 'postcode lottery of care'. The Institute's genesis can also be understood in the context of the continuing debate around whether the NHS could deliver comprehensive high quality care, free to all, or whether services would need to be prioritised or rationed (Weale, 1998). Should rationing be 'explicit' – guidelines had been mooted as a way to achieve this (Norheim, 1999); or 'implicit' – 'muddling through elegantly' as some more realistically suggested (Hunter,1998).

By December of that year the government had laid out its approach to achieving its aspirations for the NHS. The White Paper *The New NHS: Modern, Dependable* (Department of Health, 1997) described a range of organisational changes to support an underlying theme of developing national standards with the responsibility for delivering care locally (assisted by new clinical governance and audit systems).

Central to the approach was the establishment of a new National Institute for Clinical Excellence (NICE) to give a strong lead on clinical and cost-effectiveness, drawing up new guidelines and ensuring they reached all parts of the health service.

The rationale for NICE was summarised as follows:

7.10 There is a growing body of evidence on which treatments, drugs and other aspects of clinical practice are the most effective and offer best value. But it is not always easy for frontline doctors and nurses to find the evidence they need. Research results are not readily accessible and it is often difficult for busy health professionals to find their way through the proliferation of emerging guidelines, some of which are of variable quality. To ensure consistent access to beneficial care right across the NHS, the Government believes stronger arrangements are needed to promote clinical and cost effectiveness, both for drugs and other forms of treatment.

This organisation would be embedded in a new national system of monitoring organisational quality. National standards would be determined by new evidence-based National Service Frameworks (modelled on the cancer service frameworks originally proposed by Kenneth Calman, Chief Medical Officer for England in 1995 in the Calman Hine report (Calman–Hine Report, 1995)). To ensure the drive for excellence was instilled throughout the NHS, the Government also proposed a new Commission for Health Improvement.

It gave no further mention of the methods the Institute would use, but did give one hint of the preferred approach:

7.12 The National Institute's membership will be drawn from the health professions, the NHS, academics, health economists and patient interests. It will need to have access to an appropriate range of skills, including economic and managerial expertise as well as specialist input on specific issues.

The Government went on to state that it would 'consider developing the role and function of the Institute as it gathers momentum and experience'. It probably did not realise at the time how prescient that single sentence would become.

In this chapter we will first discuss the development of the clinical guidelines programme, followed by technology appraisals, and then the acquisition of new programmes. Other aspects of the Institute's mode of working will be introduced, including the emphasis on implementation, the involvement of patients and the public, and how NICE responded to the ethical challenges it faced.

Clinical guidelines

The White Paper stated:

> *7.11 A new National Institute for Clinical Excellence will be established to give new coherence and prominence to information about clinical and cost-effectiveness. It will produce and disseminate: clinical guidelines based on relevant evidence of clinical and cost-effectiveness associated clinical audit methodologies and information on good practice in clinical audit in doing so it will bring together work currently undertaken by the many professional organisations in receipt of Department of Health funding for this purpose it will work to a programme agreed with and funded from current resources by the Department of Health.*

It is interesting that the initial emphasis was on guidelines and guidance with no specific mention of 'drug technology appraisal', although the statement that 'Government believes stronger arrangements are needed to promote clinical and cost effectiveness, both for drugs and other forms of treatment' suggests something more targeted than guidelines was also envisaged.

This emphasis was not surprising as the Department of Health (DOH) had been trying for years to rationalise guidelines and ensure consistency. Historically, these had been developed by a range of institutions, including Royal Colleges, universities, and professional organisations. The White Paper highlighted that no new money would be available and the Institute would need to re-allocate money already allocated to the Royal Colleges. Initial discussions within the Institute debated the pros and cons of 'approving' selected existing guidelines, e.g. the Scottish Intercollegiate Guidelines Network (SIGN), which was already established and was supported by the English Royal College of Physicians. The then College President, Sir George Alberti, stated publicly that NICE should just endorse the SIGN guidelines. The NICE Board debated this approach, but in the end decided that a new approach to guideline development that took into account the assessment of cost-effectiveness was needed. This would require considerable resources. The decision was made to terminate all College funding for clinical audit and use it to commission a series of national collaborating centres to develop clinical guidelines.

In 2001, four such centres were established and were commissioned to develop guidelines, setting out how whole disease pathways should be approached and what standards patients should expect. They would apply the guideline development methods evolved by NICE. Independent guideline development groups were set up to include clinicians, patients, carers and other interested parties to make recommendations about the most cost-effective care. This model proved highly successful and durable, with around 300 guidelines being produced: it was only in 2022 that the approach changed and guideline development was moved inhouse within the Institute.

The original NICE methods were developed according to the principles emerging from a European Union-funded project exploring how to appraise guidelines (Cluzeau et al., 2003). This project resulted in the creation of the AGREE (Appraising Guidelines, Research and Evaluation) instrument which has since been endorsed by the European Union, the World Health Organization, and many national governments. This approach itself was based on an initial research programme in England supported by the National R&D primary/secondary interface programme. A collaboration between St Georges Medical School, Aberdeen University and St Bartholomew's Hospital Medical School resulted in the development of a critical appraisal instrument (Cluzeau et al., 1999). Subsequently St Georges was commissioned following a Europe-wide competitive tendering process to coordinate the appraisal of potential national guidelines on behalf of the NHS Executive (Cluzeau and Littlejohns, 1999).

In 2002, the first clinical guideline was published, on schizophrenia. The guideline was developed to cover the whole pathway – from diagnosis to treatment options, identifying who is responsible for the patient at every stage, and all the other aspects of care. The guideline had real impact as there was then little in the way of national guidelines for mental health. It has since been widely used, including in Australia and the state of California, and translated and adopted in Spain and Italy.

Health technology appraisals

Before NICE's establishment, in contrast to guidelines, the emphasis for drug appraisal had been at a regional level, based within commissioning structures and usually led by Public Health practitioners. A series of committees was established to identify whether new expensive drugs, mainly for cancer, should be available on the NHS. Variation in their decisions meant that there was differing availability of new drugs across the country leading to disparity in access to these drugs. News reports in which commentators walked down a street where patients on one side (in one health authority) could get a cancer drug while a similar patient on the other side (in a different health authority) could not, became common.

However, two events meant that NICE's immediate priority was to undertake the assessment of the value of single drugs. The first was that the Secretary of State Frank Dobson's attempt to limit the use of Viagra on the NHS was deemed illegal (Dyer and Bosely, 1999) (see Chapter 9) and the second was that Glaxo released its new anti-flu drug. As part of NICE's initial evaluation programme it was due to review two anti-influenza drugs, the neuraminidase inhibitors Relenza (zanamivir) and Tamiflu (oseltamivir), with a view to reporting in 2002. As this would have been too late for the pending winter flu season in Britain, NICE was asked in late 1999 to fast-track an opinion on Relenza that had been licensed in both Europe and the USA (*The Lancet*, 1999).

At this time NICE had not developed its approach to Technology Appraisals and it therefore created a bespoke rapid appraisal process. A small committee chaired by the CEO, Andrew Dillon, with the recently appointed Clinical Director, Professor Peter Littlejohns, a clinical pharmacologist, Professor Joe Collier, and clinician and ethicist Professor Ray Tallis, was to undertake the assessment. Its draft guidance would be issued for consultation. The Institute created a guidance executive to make a recommendation to the NHS on behalf of the Institute and there was to be an appeal process led by the chair of NICE, Sir Michael Rawlins. Before NICE had even formally reported on the inhalational agent zanamivir, Richard Skyes, head of Glaxo Wellcome, expressed his concern that the very idea that this drug should not be made available on the National Health Service spelled the end of an innovative British pharmaceutical industry. An 'appalled' British Pharma Group, a trio of British based global companies (the other two being Astra Zeneca and Smith Kline Beecham), wrote to the UK's prime minister on October 5 1999 to plead that NICE's verdict had 'potentially devastating consequences' (*The Lancet*, 1999).

NICE issued guidance that did not recommend its use in the NHS. The benefits were one less day of severe symptoms at a financial cost of £24 for a five day course with an estimate of £6m to £100m in an epidemic. But the real costs would be a disruption to the normal approach by GPs in watching and waiting for symptoms. If the drug were made available, patients would need to see a GP as soon as any symptoms occurred, which would overwhelm primary care services and also act as a focus for cross infection. Sykes was reported as storming into 10 Downing Street, 'incandescent'. He threatened that if the 'ludicrous' decision was not reversed, Glaxo Wellcome, then Britain's biggest pharma company, would consider leaving the UK. Briefed by Dobson, Prime Minister Tony Blair refused to overturn the decision (Yarney, 1999).

NICE proceeded quickly to set up a process of Technology Appraisal based on the principles of evidence-based medicine (EBM) and the lessons it had learnt from its first ad hoc appraisal. It was to create a system that relied on independent appraisal committees (containing a broad base of stakeholders), and open and transparent decision-making (the committees met in public). All draft guidance was consulted on, with detailed responses to all issues raised. The original appraisal committee, consisting of 30 members under the chairmanship of Professor David Barnett and deputy chair Professor Andrew Stevens, deliberated on reports developed by academic departments commissioned initially through the NHS Research Programme (and later the National Institute for Health Research), and instigated an appeal process that was based on legal principles and concepts of fairness (see Chapter 9). While originally recommendations were presented to the NHS as guidance, following pressure from the Pharma industry the Department of Health required local commissioners to make funding available for all NICE positive decisions within three months. The corollary being that a negative decision meant that the drug was not available on the NHS.

The core methods were now carefully described and updated regularly with adaptions as new programmes were established. This national approach absorbed the expertise that had previously been regionally based and these committees were closed down, ironically to re-emerge in a different guise as part of the temporary experiment with the Cancer Drugs Fund – see below.

NICE's first full technology appraisal in 2000 recommended healthy wisdom teeth should not be removed as a precaution; this was estimated to save the NHS £5m a year.

Over the next 25 years around 1,000 appraisals were undertaken. In 2006, NICE introduced a faster technology appraisal process, using a 39 week timetable, against the 54 weeks that had previously been standard.

A major challenge to the survival of NICE came in 2010 when the new Coalition government created a 'Cancer Drugs Fund' to provide access to cancer drugs that NICE had not been able to recommend, for some patients whose consultants said would nevertheless benefit from treatment (National Audit Office, 2015). This gave effect to a pledge of the new Prime Minister David Cameron in the election campaign, following lobbying by the renal cancer patient group. Many saw this as the end of the usefulness of the Institute as one of its main functions had been circumvented. However, this initiative was bedevilled by criticisms and eventually ran out of money. In 2016, new arrangements were put in place which re-focused the Fund towards providing access to cancer drugs that NICE considered had potential to benefit, but which needed more data before a final recommendation for routine use could be made. In essence, this provided funding for 'only in research' recommendations (but for cancer patients only), a third option that NICE had always had as a possibility but was never funded and so hardly used. The use of the Fund and other more recent changes to NICE's drug appraisal process meant that in some cases cancer patients could expect to access new treatments faster than in other European countries. This was a response to a recurring criticism of NICE that it slowed up access to innovative treatments. In 2016 the first drug was approved, Bosutinib, made by Pfizer for certain chronic myeloid leukaemia patients. It meant that the drug became available through normal NHS funding channels whereas previously it was only available through the Cancer Drugs Fund.

A milestone was reached at the start of 2018, when the 500th technology appraisal was published. And at the end of the same year, a breakthrough cancer treatment – called CAR T-cell therapy – for adults with certain types of non-Hodgkin lymphoma was approved for use through the new Cancer Drugs Fund. This was proposed as a possible way for the use of more personalised, innovative medicines to be accessed through the NHS.

Over time NICE expanded its technology appraisal portfolio with two new programmes to assess new medical technologies and diagnostics. It also started highly specialised technology appraisals – those that look at drugs for very rare conditions. The first recommendation was foreculizumab for a chronic, rare, progressive condition that causes severe inflammation of blood vessels and blood clots, called atypical haemolytic uraemic syndrome.

Additions to NICE's original portfolio of guidance

Over the years NICE has taken on a range of new activities. These, along with other milestones in the history of the Institute, are summarised in the box.

Timeline for the development of the Institute's work programmes

1999 National Institute for Clinical Excellence (NICE) established on 1st April
The first guidance (rapid appraisal of zanamivir) is published in October

2000 The first appraisal (TA1) on wisdom teeth is published in March

2001 The National Collaborating Centres established

2002 The first guideline (CG1) on Schizophrenia is published in December
The National Guidelines and Audit Patient Involvement Unit established (later became Public Involvement Programme within NICE)

2003 The first interventional procedures guidance (IPG1) is published on uterine artery embolisation for fibroids in July

2005 The Health Development Agency transfers to NICE
NICE becomes the National Institute for Health and Clinical Excellence

2006 The first public health guideline (PH1), smoking: brief interventions and referrals is published in March
The single technology appraisal programme started publishing guidance (to speed up the appraisal process)

2008   NICE guidance development programmes commence meetings in public

2009   NICE commences developing indicators for the Quality Outcomes Framework

NICE creates an accreditation programme for other guidance programmes

NHS Evidence launched

2010   The first quality standard (QS1) on dementia: support in health and social care is published in March

The first medical technology guidance (MTG1) is published on balloon catheters for in-stent coronary restenosis in December

2011   NICE is invited to develop indicators on behalf of the NHS Commissioning Board for the Clinical Commissioning Group Outcome Indicator set

National Prescribing Centre joins the Institute. It later became the Medicines and Prescribing Centre

NICE pathways (online tool to give access to the full range of guidelines and tools) go live

First diagnostics guidance (DG1) on the EOS2 2D/3D imaging system is published in October

2013   NICE becomes a non-departmental body

NICE takes on responsibility for developing guidance and standards in social care and changes name to National Institute for Health and Care Excellence

The NHS Technology and Adoption Centre joins NICE

2014   The first social care guidance (SC1) published on managing medicines in March

The first medicines practice guidance (MPG1) on developing and updating local formularies is published in March

2015   The first highly specialised technology guidance (HST1), eculizumab for treating haemolytic uraemic syndrome is published in January

2016   The first drug approved from old cancer drug fund, Bosulif for chronic myeloid leukaemia

Unified indicator menu launched for general practice and Clinical Commissioning Groups

NICE ceases its accreditation programme

2017   NICE issues first guidance on microbial resistance as part of a suite

2018   500th technology appraisal published

2021   NICE 2021 to 2026 strategy published with revision of methods manual

2022   Office for Digital Health launched

They include taking on functions where existing guidance development was failing to have impact, e.g. interventional procedures; where it made sense to bring guidance development together, e.g. the British National Formulary and social care; or where the guidance could be adapted for policy reasons, eg quality indicators.

Interventional procedures provides a useful case study to show how NICE took on new roles.

Globally, there are systems in place to ensure that new drugs are subjected to rigorous tests and approval before unrestricted use on patients. Medical devices are also subject to some scrutiny and approval. By contrast, approval of interventional procedures has lagged behind. Mostly undertaken by surgeons but increasingly by other specialists as well, by the late 1990s there were increasing press reports of surgical scandals and heightened public concern that led to political and patient pressure for formal systems to assess new interventions.

In the UK, initial moves were made in 1996 by setting up the Safety and Efficacy Register for New Interventional Procedures (SERNIP). It was organised by the Royal Colleges, with limited funding from the NHS, and was entirely voluntary. The register gradually accumulated a list of new procedures and allocated each to a category signifying its perceived degree of safety and efficacy. However, it soon became controversial and, following professional challenges to its assessment of new interventions for treatment of female incontinence coupled with the risk of legal challenges, the responsibility to establish a new evaluation system was transferred to NICE by the DOH in 2000. A new approach was developed and a committee established under the chairmanship of Professor Bruce Campbell.

Over the next 24 years nearly 600 interventional procedure assessments were undertaken.

The significant difference between the interventional procedures programme and other NICE programmes is that it did not assess cost-effectiveness. This was because there was little data available at the early part of the developmental cycle of these types of intervention. There was one notable exception – the assessment of the surgical prevention of variant CJD. See the box for details.

Variant CJD – a case study in the NICE approach to novel assessments

Iatrogenic Creutzfeldt-Jakob disease (CJD) may result from patient exposure to human prions through surgical or medical treatment. As a precautionary measure, single-use instruments for tonsillectomy operations were introduced in early 2001. Tonsillectomies were targeted because tonsils of affected individuals carry high levels of infective prions and also because of the young age of patients treated. In England, serious concerns about the quality of single-use instruments available for tonsillectomy and their impact on patient safety resulted in a reversal of this decision less than a year later and the re-introduction of re-usable instruments for all tonsillec-tomies. In Wales, however, following the establishment of quality control systems, single-use instruments continued to be used for tonsillectomies, and relevant complication rates were no higher than those of reusable ones. Balancing the patient safety implications from potentially substand-ard single-use instruments against the risk of transmission of variant CJD (vCJD) via reusable instruments became a constant challenge faced by policy-makers in this field.

In May 2004, the Chief Medical Officer (CMO) for England, on behalf of all UK CMOs, invited NICE to develop and publish guidance to the NHS on how best to manage the risk of transmission of CJD and variant CJD via interventional procedures. The initial referral was to look at effectiveness only. However, debate between the senior staff at NICE, with the Clinical Director advocating the importance of value for money assessments of such a far-reaching decision, resulted in this view prevailing, and the referral became one of assessing cost-effectiveness. The guidance would consider more than 2 million procedures under-taken in the UK every year, involving a wide range of tissues that could potentially transmit CJD. It would apply to all patients undergoing these procedures excluding those thought to be at risk of carrying the dis-ease, for whom relevant DOH guidelines should be applied. It would be the first guidance addressing such a wide range of patients and surgical procedures.

NICE set up a bespoke process, merging elements of its health tech-nology appraisal and interventional procedure programmes. Following two rounds of public consultation the guidance was published in Novem-ber 2006.

To develop the guidance, the Institute convened a panel of experts who formed the CJD Advisory Sub-Committee (CJDAS). CJDAS con-sisted of clinicians, scientists, epidemiologists, health economists, gov-ernment agency representatives and a lay member. Several members of CJDAS, including its Chair (Bruce Campbell), were practising surgeons. Practical input from frontline clinicians familiar with the operating thea-tre environment ensured the guidance was realistic and implementable in an NHS setting. Clinical involvement was not limited to the Sub-Committee membership. The views of professional bodies were actively sought and influenced the final recommendations through the two rounds of consultation and specialist advice. To assist the Sub-Committee in its task, NICE commissioned an independent academic group (the Review Group) to undertake a systematic review of the literature and produce a risk assessment, that is, to try and quantify the risk of transmission of

CJD via interventional procedures based on the existing evidence. Having modelled more than 2 million procedures, and based on the levels of risk and associated costs, the Sub-Committee decided to focus on those procedures that were considered to carry a high risk for CJD transmission: those in ophthalmic surgery, operations on retina and optic nerve and in neurosurgery, and intradural operations on the brain, including neuroendoscopy.

The guidance

Three main measures were considered as means of reducing the risk of transmission of CJD by the Committee: (i) introduction of safe and more effective decontamination methods; (ii) elimination of migration of instruments between sets; and (iii) introduction of single-use instruments.

See here for more details of process and guidance https://www.ncbi.nlm.nih.gov/pmc/articles/PMC1963552/

In 2005, and as discussed further in Chapter 7, issuing Public Health guidance became part of NICE's remit as it absorbed the Health Development Agency which was producing guidelines intended to ensure healthier lives – on breastfeeding, falls prevention, smoking cessation and healthy schools. NICE changed its name to the National Institute for Health and Clinical Excellence (the acronym remained the same).

Further changes occurred in 2013 as NICE became a non-departmental public body, enabling it to provide guidelines for the social care sector. This wider remit was reflected in a further change to name, and NICE became the National Institute for Health and Care Excellence. In March 2014, the first social care guidance was issued outlining how medicines in care homes should be managed. Over the next nine years, 71 guidance documents aimed specifically at social care were developed.

The core principle of NICE was that it based its guidance on the best available evidence. What 'best available' means is an important element as many 'pure EBMers' felt that unless there was 'gold standard' evidence (e.g. randomised control trials), guidance should not be issued. NICE laid out its approach in a range of papers (Littlejohns et al., 2009) but the debate continues. In later years, as well as using evidence, NICE also became involved in summarising data and information. In 2009, NHS Evidence (which later became the Evidence Service) was launched. It created a unified evidence base for everyone in the NHS who made decisions about treatments or the use of resources, and for patients who wanted to know more about their care. Its creation heralded the start of NICE providing a suite of additional services and resources to support evidence-based decision-making in health and social care, including Clinical Knowledge summaries for primary care.

NICE values

As it started to produce its appraisal guidance and negative decisions were generating increasing public debate, government advisors were anxious that NICE should take steps to ensure that the general public understood the need for prioritisation and how NICE did it. NICE responded in two ways. First, by establishing a Citizens Council in 2002 (Littlejohns and Rawlins 2009), which provided a public perspective on the moral and ethical issues that NICE should take into account when producing guidance. The Council's recommendations and conclusions have informed NICE's methodology. Interestingly this was run as part of the Institute's R&D programme under the leadership of the Clinical Director rather than in the Institute's Patient and Involvement Programme.

A representative panel of 30 members of the public, the Citizens Council was an innovative way to bring the voice of the public into the guidance that NICE produces. Its first report stated that NICE should not consider whether a disease or a condition was 'self-induced' when deciding on what care to provide. In addition to the Citizens Council, the Institute worked closely with patients and the public to ensure their involvement in guidance development. This aspect of its work is discussed in more detail in Chapter 8.

The second approach was to be clear on the values that underpinned all of NICE's decisions. In 2005 the NICE R&D programme developed its *Social Value Judgements* document, subsequently updated in 2008 (NICE, 2008). In addition to this, in January 2009, NICE introduced new criteria for drugs that provide additional benefit at the end of life. A groundswell of public opinion and some evidence that society places extra value on the weeks and months at the end of life for terminally ill patients led to NICE introducing a higher threshold for those drugs that could extend life for patients whose life expectancy was two years or less. However, in 2020 NICE moved away from social values to creating more process driven values. This change of direction is explored in depth in several of the chapters in this book (see Chapters 4, 5 and 6).

Why the book?

The publication of *Social Value Judgements* was reflective of a recognition on the part of NICE that the evidence which was collected could not simply be mechanically applied to yield a particular recommendation. Rather, members of the Institute's committees would need to apply their skills, knowledge and experience to reach the necessary conclusions. The document identified the types of judgement required as being of two varieties: 'scientific value judgements are about interpreting the quality and significance of the evidence available; social value judgements relate to society rather than science' (NICE, 2008: 4).

This provides an important insight into the broad reach of NICE's role, and the diversity of understandings required of those who work for it, beyond the immediate clinical, public health and social care arena in which it operated. The Institute's methodologies, processes and outputs have necessarily made use of, and themselves influenced, a disparate range of disciplinary approaches and evidence. This has extended well beyond 'pure' science and, accordingly, generated interest from a wide variety of scholars from across the domain of the social sciences; and it is this breadth of disciplinary engagement which provides the motivation for this book.

Most obviously, economics sits at the heart of NICE decision-making. Law provides the framework within which the Institute is required to exercise its functions, and a means of holding it to account. As a regulatory body, NICE can be seen as an exemplar of modern developments in governance, thus drawing the attention of those working in political science. Its authority – legitimacy – to make difficult choices, especially in its health technology appraisal work, has been scrutinised by political theorists. The moral issues underpinning those choices, which raise fundamental questions of distributive justice, are a matter of concern to philosophers and ethicists. Sociologists seek to understand the internal organisational dynamics of the Institute, the role of patients and the public in its decision-making, and its impact upon population health inequalities. No doubt this list could be extended, both as regards topics and disciplines.

This book seeks to mark the Institute's 25th anniversary by drawing upon a number of these wider social science approaches to explore various dimensions of, and controversial issues arising from, NICE's work in the health context over the past 25 years, as well as certain of its successes and failures in that period. As noted previously, it is not intended to offer a comprehensive history of the Institute, although inevitably some of the contributions address aspects of its historical development. Rather, the goal is to present a varied collection of disciplinary perspectives which, it is hoped, will provide readers with a fuller understanding of the evolution of this important and durable institution, and to afford some insights into how it might respond to the challenges it might face in the future.

First, in Chapter 2, health economists Karl Claxton, Mark Sculpher and Anthony Culyer describe the evolution over time of the methods and processes of health technology assessment, and the implications of such developments for NICE's health care mission.

In Chapter 3, David J. Hunter and Peter Littlejohns consider reasons for the longevity of NICE, a highly notable phenomenon in the rapidly changing British regulatory landscape (especially within the NHS). Using models derived from political science, they analyse the political context in which NICE functioned and the factors and strategies which enabled it to survive.

Public policy expert and political theorist Albert Weale critically considers NICE as a case-study in public practical reasoning in Chapter 4. He discusses the meaning and ethical appropriateness of the 'classical paradigm' of NICE decision-making, rooted in utilitarianism and welfare economics. The chapter analyses whether the Institute's recent move from 'values' to 'principles' represents a shift in this paradigm, or not.

The issue of whether the character of NICE decision-making has changed over time is pursued further in Chapter 5. Victoria Charlton draws on insights from empirical bioethics to explore how NICE's normative approach has evolved over time, and what this might mean for the legitimacy of its societal role.

The increasing importance of innovation in the work of NICE, a topic explored in the previous two chapters (and in Chapter 2), also informs Chapter 6. Here, philosopher James Wilson explores whether this focus, and NICE's approach to assessment of highly specialised technologies, can plausibly be said to lead to an overall improvement in the services that the NHS provides.

Moving beyond health care, in Chapter 7, Michael P. Kelly, formerly Director of the Centre for Public Health Excellence at NICE, discusses the work of NICE in developing evidence-based guidelines on cost-effective public health interventions and programmes. He analyses the methodological innovations, the practical problems, and the political controversies which arose as a consequence of NICE's involvement in this field.

In Chapter 8, Sophie Staniszewska and Sophie Söderholm Werkö describe how the Institute involved patients and the public in its decision-making processes from its very inception, and how this activity has evolved over time.

Recognising the role which legal intervention in resource allocation played in NICE's establishment, in Chapter 9 Keith Syrett describes the challenges which confronted NICE in the courtroom, and analyses judicial responses to its decision-making. More broadly, he considers what this demonstrates as to the assumed role for law in the contemporary 'regulatory state', and whether legal oversight has contributed to NICE's attainment of legitimacy.

In Chapter 10, Ryan Jonathan Sitanggang, Kinanti Khansa Chavarina, Kalipso Chalkidou, Fiona Pearce and Yot Teerawattananon assess the influence and impact of NICE on the international health technology assessment landscape. They also discuss the work of NICE International.

Finally, in Chapter 11, Peter Littlejohns, David J. Hunter and Keith Syrett, drawing on analysis presented in the preceding chapters, identify common themes and features that enabled NICE to thrive. The chapter also looks to the future, identifying certain of the challenges which NICE will face moving into the next quarter-century of its existence, and what it might need to do to survive.

References

Calman–Hine Report (1995) *A Report by the Expert Advisory Group on Cancer to the Chief Medical Officers of England and Wales. A Policy Framework for Commissioning Cancer Services*. London: Department of Health.
Cluzeau, F., Littlejohns, P., Grimshaw, J., Feder, G. and Moran S.E. (1999) 'Development and application of a generic methodology to assess the quality of clinical guidelines', *International Journal for Quality in Health Care*, 11(1), pp.21–28.

Cluzeau, F. and Littlejohns, P. (1999) 'Appraising clinical practice guidelines in England and Wales: the development of a methodological framework and its application in policy', *Joint Commission Journal on Quality Improvement*, 25(10), pp.514–21.

Cluzeau, F., Burgers, J., Brouwers, M., Grol, R., Mäkelä, M., Littlejohns, P., Grimshaw, J. and Hunt, C. (2003) 'Development and validation of an international appraisal instrument for assessing the quality of clinical practice guidelines: the AGREE project', *Quality and Safety in Health Care*, 12, pp.18–23.

Department of Health (1997) *The New NHS Modern, Dependable*. Cm 3807, London: The Stationery Office.

Dyer, C. and Bosely, S. (1999) 'Viagra rationing "unlawful"', *The Guardian* (27 May). Available at: https://www.theguardian.com/uk/1999/may/27/claredyer.sarahboseley (Accessed 12 October 2023).

Hunter, D.J. (1998) *Desperately Seeking Solutions: Rationing Health Care*. London: Routledge.

The Lancet (1999) 'A nasty start for NICE', *The Lancet*, 354(9187), p.1313.

Littlejohns P., Chalkidou, K., Wyatt, J. and Pearson, S. (2009) 'Assessing evidence and prioritizing clinical and public health guidance recommendations: the NICE way', in Killoran, A. and Kelly, M.P., *Evidence-based Public Health: Effectiveness and Efficiency*. Oxford: Oxford University Press, pp.326–34.

Littlejohns, P. and Rawlins, M. (eds) (2009) *Patients, the Public and Priorities in Health Care*. Oxford: Radcliffe.

National Audit Office (2015) *Investigation into the Cancer Drugs Fund*. HC 442 (2015–16).

NICE (2008) *Social Value Judgements: Principles for the Development of NICE Guidance*. 2nd edn. London: NICE.

Norheim, O.F. (1999) 'Healthcare rationing—are additional criteria needed for assessing evidence based clinical practice guidelines?', *British Medical Journal*, 319(7222), pp.1426–29.

Weale, A. (1998) 'Rationing health care', *British Medical Journal*, 316(7129), p.410.

Yarney, G. (1999) 'NICE to rule on influenza flu drug zanamivir', *British Medical Journal*, 319(7215), p.942a.

2 NICE and resource allocation in the NHS

Paradise lost?

Karl Claxton, Mark Sculpher and Anthony J. Culyer

NICE – a promise of paradise?

In the formative years of NICE from 1998 on, the hopes of many supporters, including the three of us, were ambitious; perhaps crazily so. The National Institute for Clinical Excellence (NICE) was created to provide clear standards based on clinical- and cost-effectiveness, resolve uncertainty about appropriate treatment modes, minimise inappropriate variation in clinical practice, and to promote faster uptake of cost-effective treatments and more equitable access to cost-effective treatments and care. In the 1990s the idea of clinical governance was in vogue: a framework through which NHS organizations are accountable for continually improving the quality of their services and safeguarding high standards of care by creating an environment in which excellence in clinical care will flourish. NICE was to provide the evidential underpinning for clinical governance. For us, NICE was also to be the central model of how to run an NHS that would be fairer (no postcode rationing), well-delivered by clinicians, well-informed, well-managed, well-understood by all (from top politicians of all parties to the humblest citizen), still free at the point of use, one that did not pay manufacturers over the top for its medicines, and one that maximised the impact of its resources on the health of the people. More generally (this is the crazy bit,) it was to be a model for other parts of the public sector, with substitution of appropriate departmental objectives: social care, educational attainment, national security, fair and speedy access to justice, adequate housing, international aid. This would contribute to a more informed and evidence-based public debate about the appropriate scale and allocation of public expenditure, thereby strengthening the social democratic process itself.

How were such beliefs possible? Some critical factors were in place:

- We shared a common belief that economics as a social science also had a social purpose, which was to serve the public good.
- We shared a common belief that, whatever our own preferences might be, the public good was not for us to define, let alone determine.

DOI: 10.4324/9781003501268-2

- We shared a common belief that economics served the public interest in health best in alliance with other approaches, most notably evidence-based medicine, epidemiology, and public health.
- We shared a common belief that the technical tools required for NICE to serve the public good were substantially to hand.
- We were eager for a suitable application to demonstrate the practical value of economics' social purpose.
- We shared a common belief that the process of decision-making required the active participation of all important stakeholders.

The social purpose of NICE was defined politically: to remove inequalities (specifically, the regional variations in the area availability of services and differences in clinical practice termed 'postcode prescribing') and to establish evidence-informed best practice norms in the clinical use of medical interventions of all kinds (especially medicines). These objectives were set by the Secretary of State for Health, not by the occupants of academic ivory towers.

The potential of well-designed interdisciplinary collaboration had been amply demonstrated through numerous applications of the methods of economic evaluation, most notably, cost-effectiveness analysis, on which, by 1998, there was a substantial published literature in professional journals, both specialist and multi-disciplinary. NICE's chair, Mike Rawlins, was a convinced supporter of the principles on which an explicit assessment of cost-effectiveness is founded and wanted NICE from the start to be authoritative in this regard.

Many of the tools for empirical analysis were already available or under development, including randomised clinical trials; the collection of resource use/cost data; cost-effectiveness analysis; decision analytic modelling; a growing capacity for conducting systematic reviews, evidence synthesis and meta-analysis; a generic measure of health outcome (the quality-adjusted life-year or QALY); methods for quantifying and communicating uncertainty and the value of additional research; budget management methods such as programme budgeting. There were also some key concepts, whose practical measurement would be challenging, of which the most important by far was the idea of 'opportunity cost': the health that could have been gained had the additional resources required to accommodate a new technology been made available to the NHS with existing technologies.

The need for a participatory approach to decision-making was not simply the obvious one of multi-disciplinarity and multi-professionality, it was also seen as one means of generating relevant evidence and of testing the relevance and acceptability of many of the value judgments that were intrinsically involved. We did not favour deliberative participation solely for its own sake. Deliberation and participation were needed also for instrumental reasons. In specific cases, crucial evidence, for example, was available only from the manufacturers of the product being evaluated; it was not expected that the QALY (as it then was) would serve reliably as a single indicator and would need to be tested in specific circumstances against the experience of people with the condition in question, family carers and others with vicarious experience; effective methods of communicating decisions and the reasons would require skills in academic, professional and 'lay' presentation. Participation was also needed in the process by which topics for specific investigation were to be selected and at various points in the development of specific clinical guidelines and technology appraisals (see Chapter 8).

The years of hope

Better decisions with better methods

NICE was not the first example of a public body formally using economic evaluation to help define appropriate clinical practice. Such an approach had been used in Australia from 1992 (Commonwealth Department of Health, 1992) and the Canadian province of Ontario since 1994 (Ministry of Health, 1994). It was, however, the NHS' first foray at a national level into the development of routine evidence-based guidance with economic evaluation front and centre. Importantly, NICE's views on appropriate methods were defined at an early stage (NICE, 1999). They reflected best practice internationally in the applied economic evaluation of health care technologies. A firm position was taken on the need for a generic measure of health to facilitate comparison across diseases and types of intervention, not least to enable a comparison of the health benefits offered with the likely health opportunity costs which would fall on other patients with a range of different conditions. For these reasons the widely used QALY was adopted within a cost-effectiveness framework.

The emphasis on costs falling on the NHS (rather than the broader public sector or wider economy) was also the defined focus at this stage. This 'narrow' perspective was consistent with NICE's remit as a special health authority, although this drew pushback from some economists that a 'societal' viewpoint should be adopted notwithstanding the challenges of its implementation. Another key feature of NICE's early methods position was to eschew a rigid definition of 'valid' evidence of relevant outcomes. The evidence-based medicine movement had focussed more or less exclusively on randomised clinical trials (RCTs) to establish clinical effectiveness, with stringent criteria to define quality. Whilst RCTs were to be central to NICE's decision-making, an early commitment was to review all relevant evidence, to understand its strengths and limitations, and to reflect the implications of key uncertainties for decision-making throughout the economic evaluation.

A further important feature of NICE's early approach was the use of 'third-party' analysts (academic assessment groups), independent of the Institute and its appraisal committees, as the primary means by which relevant evidence was identified, synthesised and modelled. Submissions from technology manufacturers were a key source of evidence and generally included their own systematic reviews and economic evaluations, but the assessment groups were given time to develop their own analyses, informed by the manufactuers' evidence. These early appraisals were scoped to include as many new proprietary technologies as necessary for a relevant clinical indication, with the purpose of providing clarity to the NHS on which, if any, available interventions were recommended for funding, a process later defined as multiple technology assessment (MTA).

A major step forward in defining NICE's methods and approaches to decision-making was made in the 2004 *Guide to the Methods of Technology Appraisal* (NICE, 2004). The process of generating this more granular definition of NICE's chosen methods involved a range of stakeholders (academic, clinical, NHS, industry), and sought to apply the principles of good science to NHS decisions. The concept of the 'reference case' economic analysis was adopted as suggested by the first Panel on Cost-Effectiveness in Health and Medicine (Gold et al., 1996). This reflected the need for consistent methods to support decisions, and allowed appropriate deviations in methods when these could be clearly justified. Prominence and clarity were given to the role of decision analytic modelling, methods for capturing uncertainty, the development of the EQ-5D 3L as the standard QALY measure and extrapolating clinical evidence beyond short-term Randomized Controlled Trials (RCTs).

NICE also formed a greater understanding of the challenging ethical issues that lie at the heart of decisions about the allocation of collective resources in health (see Chapter 5). It had rightly understood that these could not be resolved with technical remedies marshalled by academics, but needed contributions from the wider public (see Chapter 8). To this end, the establishment of the NICE Citizens Council in 2002 was an important step in building authority and confidence in its decision-making (Littlejohns and Rawlins, 2009). The Council was a group of approximately 30 members of the public, broadly representative of the UK population, which considered early topics including clinical need (NICE Citizens Council, 2002) and the rule of rescue (NICE Citizens Council, 2006).

The advent of NICE, its commitment to evidence and analysis of economic value as well as clinical effectiveness, generated important partnerships and collaboration in the UK. The assessment groups developed their own grouping (InterTASC) which provided a forum for discussing methods. A group of methodologists working in Technology Assessment Review (TAR) groups and active on the NICE Appraisal Committee supported NICE with challenging evidence and methods questions. An early application came in NICE's first appraisal of new drug treatments for multiple sclerosis (MS) in 2002 (Chilcott et al., 2003). This was problematic in terms of the available evidence and the modelling necessary to quantity clinical benefits and cost-effectiveness. The group used novel methods to characterise the natural history of MS and to model the benefits of the new drugs, which was fundamental to NICE's initial guidance. The funding of this group's work showed NICE's early commitment to working with the best in the field to address complex and highly politicised challenges. The group working on MS became the first incarnation of the NICE Decision Support Unit (DSU) which provided methods support after 2005 in areas as diverse as survival modelling, weighting QALYs and evidence synthesis.

NICE and deliberation

Deliberative processes are frequently characterised as participatory and interactive methods for explicitly and systematically combining different types of evidence. However, around the time of NICE's launch, there existed no widely accepted concept, no clear statement of its scope, and little guidance as to the institutional forms it would ideally take that would distinguish it from mere consultation and opportunities for interested parties to comment, for example, on drafts of decisions. NICE took an ad hoc approach. We saw the necessity of involving a sufficient range of stakeholders for NICE to be visibly impartial and credible.

There were several reasons why deliberation needed to be at the heart of NICE's processes:

- Good policy guidance requires the combination of heterogeneous evidence, qualitative and quantitative, reliable and unreliable, with known and unknown biases, oral and written. Combining all these would require thoughtful meetings, good briefing, good chairing, and opportunities for discussion and debate. The biggest challenge would be the combining of cost and outcome information with the use of professional judgments ('colloquial' evidence) based on practice experience alongside 'harder' scientific epidemiological evidence from clinical and other trials.
- This seemed an attractive form of democratic governance, being tied to public involvement and engagement, both for its own sake and to increase the legitimacy, accountability, credibility and acceptability of decisions.
- It needed authority in making its scientific judgements (as assessed by scientists) and its social value judgements (as assessed by other stakeholders), both of which could be controversial.
- It needed to demonstrate humanity by manifestly understanding the concerns of patients, families and caregivers, and of the wider public.
- This would provide a means through which gaps in knowledge could be identified by participating stakeholders and inputs thereby provided for future NICE-relevant research.
- Deliberation could generate new evidence, for example in the form of summarized views of public preferences, values and perspectives: 'colloquial' evidence.

NICE created National Collaborating Centres (NCCs) in collaboration with the Royal Medical Colleges for clinical guideline development. Each NCC was a professionally led group with the experience and resources to develop clinical guidance for the NHS. Each NCC would define the scope of the guideline and create a guideline development group consisting of health professionals, lay representatives and technical experts. Consultees could comment on the draft guideline, to be posted on the NICE website during two consultation periods. A review panel would review the guideline, check that stakeholder comments had been addressed, and validate the final guideline.

For appraisals of technologies, standing appraisal committees with members (unpaid) appointed for a three-year term were drawn from the NHS, patient/ caregiver organizations, relevant academic disciplines and the pharmaceutical and medical devices industries. Members' names were posted on NICE's website. The appraisal committees were deliberative. They received special systematic reviews of the technologies under investigation and economic evaluations by the assessment groups and submissions from stakeholder groups. Their final appraisal determination, the basis of advice to the NHS, would be appealable. In these early years NICE was willing to see controversial decisions tested on appeal and ultimately at judicial review (see Chapter 9). For example, the 2002 decision to reject drugs for multiple sclerosis patients as not cost-effective was appealed, but the Appraisal Committee and NICE sustained its original guidance. It was the Department of Health that decided to provide access through a risk sharing agreement with manufacturers, which failed to deliver the rebates promised, conditional on the evidence that was gathered (McCabe et al., 2010). This experience may explain the later reluctance to consider anything other than more simple discounts during appraisal.

Another important milestone in these early years was the controversial guidance in 2006 to restrict access to products for Alzheimer's disease, judging their use in early or late stage disease as not cost-effective (Dyer, 2006). NICE sustained this guidance through the appeal process and it was ultimately tested at judicial review (see Chapter 9). Importantly, the outcome of judicial review validated the use of the principles of cost-effectiveness analysis, founded on decision analytic modelling, and the use of QALYs as the primary metric of health benefit. At this point, NICE process and methods had been fully tested in a number of technically and politically challenging appraisals and not found to be wanting. The independence of the Appraisal Committees and the courage of NICE to defend the principles that underpinned its guidance appeared to be assured.

International impact

These early years were characterised by a clarity in NICE's mission and rapid development and implementation of methods of clinical and economic evaluation to support decisions. These developments were recognised internationally (see Chapter 10). In the 1980s and 1990s there had been a loose collaboration of researchers working in economic evaluation of health care, but as a melting pot of disciplines including public health, economics and policy analysis. A feature of this community was its multi-disciplinarity and focus on supporting decisions on the allocation of collective resources. It had a range of intellectual influences including normative contributions from applied welfare economics.

This loose association of researchers had been publishing applied economic evaluations since the mid-1970s; some of which were used to inform important policy decisions, including some in the UK (e.g., Buxton and colleagues' economic analysis of the emerging NHS heart transplantation service in the early 1980s (Buxton et al., 1985)). Australia and Ontario's use of these methods to support drug coverage decisions gave further impetus to this emerging science. However, the centrality of economic evaluation in the new NICE technology appraisal programme represented a step change in the visibility of and interest in these methods. It brought the field's methods questions, such as the suitability of the QALY and the evidential basis of NICE's cost-effectiveness threshold range, to a wider audience which included readers of its extensive coverage in the mainstream media. Over time, many other countries developed so-called 'health technology assessment' organisations with formal methods of economic evaluation at their core and many (e.g., Ireland, Portugal, New Zealand) used NICE's documentation as a template.

As well as a validation of the relevance of many people's research over decades, the advent of NICE highlighted the need for further methods developments in areas such as quantifying uncertainty, reflecting equity considerations and conducting empirical research on the opportunity costs of decisions. A crucial concept lying at the heart of economic evaluation in health care is opportunity cost: the forgone health when resources are deployed from one use to another or when new resources are used in one particular way rather than another. The health benefit that is likely to be forgone is then compared with the health gain from the new use. While central to cost-effectiveness in health services, this fundamental 'truth' was not fully grasped by NICE after about 2005.

Paradise lost

NICE losing its way

It is important to acknowledge the significant growth over this period in the politicisation of everything NICE does and publishes (see Chapter 3). NICE has clearly had to cope with inconsistent (and often incoherent) policies from different parts of government, including changes in (the growth of) its budget alongside a growing workload. The complexities of the political environment in which NICE operates are limited in their transparency. Here no attempt is made to describe that environment or to judge the appropriateness of NICE's responses; we aim only to characterise the implications of some of the key changes that NICE has initiated.

There had, from the beginning, been some opposition to the new methods of technology appraisal which were robustly defended by the academic community (Claxton and Culyer, 2006; Ferner, Hughes and Aronson, 2010). After the mid 'noughties', however, NICE's responses to external criticism tended to retreat from the principles embodied in its early approaches to process, methods and evidence. One important development was the move in 2008 from multiple to single technology assessments (MTAs to STAs). This entailed the evaluation of individual technologies (invariably drugs) with the main evidence, presentation, synthesis and assessment provided by a product's manufacturer and the 'third party' assessment taking the form of a review by an Evidence Review Group (ERG). This change was made despite an understanding that manufacturers' results were often more optimistic than those of the assessment groups (Miners et al., 2005). In many cases, the companies' models and presentation of evidence fell short of best practice, but there was little scope for the ERGs to address these weaknesses, because they were generally limited to doing no more than further sensitivity analyses and requesting changes by the manufacturers to which they did not always respond. The consequence was, in general, weaker scrutiny of the evidence before it reached the Appraisal Committee, and a diminished evaluative framework for the Committee's deliberations and decisions. The one-at-a-time STA process was also inherently doomed to generate guidance that became outdated sooner than that of more comprehensive comparative appraisals.

STAs were certainly faster than MTAs but had a material effect on the evidential bases of NICE decisions which had been so impactful in the early years. It would have been preferable to have set criteria for prioritising technologies for assessment (e.g., scale of usage, number of technologies relevant to the indication, budget impact, potential population health effects), tailoring the assessment process for each product accordingly. A further, little discussed, consequence of moving to STAs is the effective disappearance from technology appraisal of important therapeutic medical devices if they are not expected to be cost neutral or cost saving, and which had been included in the MTA process.

Rather than developing greater sophistication in its methods of analysis and building on its founding principles, NICE increasingly made *ad hoc* adjustments (not on an evidential basis) and concessions, seemingly, to give some types of intervention an 'easier ride' through appraisal. A prominent example of this was the introduction of NICE's end of life criteria in 2009 (Bovenberg, Penton and Buyukkaramikli, 2021), which effectively gave extra weight to the benefits of drugs for patients with very short life expectancy by raising the NICE cost-effectiveness approval threshold. The stated justification was that this was an appropriate public equity consideration for these high need patients, although this was not an evidenced belief. Further, in 2022 NICE changed its methods to 'equity weight' for disease severity rather than short life expectancy alone, again, with scant regard for evidence (NICE, 2022).

Decisions for new drugs for patients with very rare diseases have also been an area where NICE has relaxed its criteria (see Chapter 6). Funding decisions for these products has been a challenge for the NHS for some time, and it was only in 2013 that NICE took responsibility for guidance for this category of products through its Highly Specialised Technologies (HST) programme. Although the criteria for a new product being appraised under HST are stringent, the assessment of value for money is relaxed compared to the main technology appraisal programme. The cost-effectiveness approval threshold under HST is £100,000 per additional QALY, compared with £20,000–30,000/QALY for the main appraisal programme, which may be increased to £300,000/QALY for large gains in health outcome (NICE, 2017). Again, there is little evidence to suggest the public view disease rarity as an attribute deserving additional priority in resource allocation decisions (Gu et al., 2023). Indeed, NICE's own Citizens Council report on ultra-orphan diseases was split on whether rarity should be a priority attribute (NICE Citizens Council, 2004).

NICE failed to explain how these various equity characteristics fitted its consideration of opportunity cost. From its early days, NICE was clear that decisions to fund more costly newer technologies should generate health improvements for those receiving the new interventions that exceeded the opportunity costs for (anonymous) NHS patients in the form of the opportunity for health gain lost through reduced services elsewhere. Although the *principle* of opportunity costs has always been embraced by NICE, the reflection in its methods and processes has been limited to a vague link to its cost-effectiveness approval thresholds. However, the patient characteristics of short life expectancy and having a rare disease to which NICE has given additional 'equity weights' are also present amongst the wider group of NHS patients. The implied ethical requirement to weight their opportunity costs appropriately escaped notice (anonymity again implying irrelevance).

NICE's specific choice of cost-effectiveness thresholds had been controversial from the beginning. It was, of course, arbitrary, reflecting values implied by decisions made prior to 2004 (Rawlins and Culyer, 2004). But it was set as a generous range, to permit use of other criteria than cost-effectiveness alone (NICE never espoused a single criterion), and to gather evidence over time as to whether the range was too permissive (i.e. admitting more procedures than the NHS budget could support) or too tight (i.e. not admitting relatively cost-effective procedures) (Culyer et al., 2007).

NICE and others (e.g., the House of Commons Health Committee, 2008) recommended the commissioning in 2009 of research by the Medical Research Council to develop an empirical basis for its cost-effectiveness threshold (Longworth et al., 2011). This research was duly commissioned and was first reported in 2013 (involving two of the authors of this chapter) (Claxton et al.,

2013; Claxton, Martin et al., 2015). It estimated the opportunity cost of additional financial costs falling on the NHS – in effect, the marginal productivity of the system. Its central estimate was that every £13,000 increase (decrease) in NHS expenditure would increase (decrease) population health outcomes by one QALY. Subsequent research, using more recent data and alternative methods, generated similar results (Lomas, Martin and Claxton, 2019; Martin et al., 2021). A measure of health opportunity cost of £15,000/QALY based on this work is routinely used in health impact analyses undertaken by the Department of Health and Social Care – for example (Department of Health, 2017).

Despite the importance (in principle) of opportunity cost in NICE's founding purpose and much of its justification for assessing the cost-effectiveness of new technologies, this evidence on health opportunity cost has not been used by NICE in any form. Various options were available to NICE to use opportunity cost evidence in the assessment and appraisal process, but none was adopted. An important implication of this is that, viewed from a public health perspective where everyone's health is considered equally, NICE's decisions on new technologies can only have reduced overall population health. Again, the costs fall on anonymous citizens (see Chapter 6). Out of sight, unrepresented in the process, and therefore out of mind.

Implications

This growing body of empirical evidence of the scale and nature of the likely opportunity costs of NICE guidance suggests that the scale of that harm is considerable. Indeed, rather than NICE being the guardian of all NHS patients, who should count and be accounted for in a principled and evidence-based way, NICE could quite reasonably be viewed as the key mechanism for manufacturers gaining access to the NHS and being able to achieve sales volumes for products, despite these being unaffordable at a local level. Central to this mechanism was the funding requirement attached to NICE guidance early in its history, which ensured that any technology receiving NHS approval must be made available at a local level. This was initially regarded by many as a positive development, reflecting confidence in NICE appraisal at the highest level, ensuring that evidence-based guidance would have an impact on what was made available to patients and was an important mechanism to ensure an end to post-code prescribing.

All this may have been true if NICE guidance did indeed reflect what was affordable at a local level. However, the weight of empirical and anecdotal evidence suggests that it did not and that the health opportunity costs of accommodating NHS guidance exceeded the health benefits to some considerable extent. A conservative view of the likely scale of harm to benefit ratio when NICE approves a new technology at £30,000 per QALY is in the region of 3 to 1. Indeed, recent evidence suggests that the health opportunity costs in areas of higher mortality are likely to be even greater (Martin et al., 2022). This means that national guidance currently increases health inequalities (Love-Koh et al., 2020). Nor does the imposition of national guidance reduce variation in access to effective health care. It does reduce variation for those patients who might benefit from those technologies approved by NICE, but it inevitably leads to differential access to the health care which must be curtailed to accommodate it.

As early as 2004, NICE was urged to move away from expressing cost-effectiveness as a comparison of an incremental costs effectiveness ratio with a 'threshold', and instead simply report an evidence-based assessment of the health benefits alongside the likely health opportunity costs (Claxton, 2008). Later, when considering value-based assessment, which included an assessment of severity and wider social benefits for the wider economy, NICE was urged to represent this, not as a change in the 'threshold' it would apply in different circumstances, but as a comparison of the range of benefits gained alongside the same range of benefits likely to be forgone due to the additional NHS costs (Claxton, Sculpher et al., 2015). The Appraisal Committee could then consider whether or not any net health loss from approving a drug was compensated for by the severity of disease or any net gains in wider social benefits. More recently NICE has returned to these considerations, but again, prefers to dial up the 'threshold' it will apply in certain circumstances, rather than clearly set out the types of health benefits gained and lost.

The need to support incentives for innovation has been cited for some time as one justification for applying 'thresholds' that do not reflect the likely health opportunity costs (Kennedy, 2009). However, the recent evidence of the long-term value of a sample of technologies approved by NICE suggests that, for most products, the net harm done during the patent period is not compensated for by cheaper generic versions in the future (Woods et al., 2021) (see Chapter 5). This means that NICE guidance is often giving away more than 100% of the long term value of an innovation in payments to manufacturers. As well as causing short and long term net harm by approving the use of these technologies, NICE guidance is also incentivising the development of future innovations at prices and manufacturing costs, which will also do long term net harm to the NHS (Woods et al., 2022).

A similar reluctance to embrace methods which clearly expose evidence-based trade-offs is evident in how NICE considers uncertainty, even though consideration of uncertainty and the need for additional research were one of its five founding principles. As noted above, NICE has quite rightly taken a broad view of relevant evidence and, when issuing guidance, has focused on expected costs and health benefits. However, such an inclusive approach must also include an evidence-based assessment of the consequences of uncertainty to the NHS (Claxton, Sculpher and Drummond, 2002). Although uncertainty is reflected in the methods of appraisal, it is not used to identify the health benefits of reducing it through additional research, nor does it identify the price reduction that would be required to compensate for this weakness (Claxton and Sculpher, 2006; Griffin et al., 2011). Nor is the assessment of the benefits of additional evidence linked to the possibility of NICE restricting use until more evidence is provided and uncertainties are resolved (Claxton, Palmer et al., 2012; Longworth et al., 2013). The risk here is that NICE issues guidance based on very uncertain estimates of the long-term costs and benefits, but that these technologies are quickly diffused into the NHS and the prospects of being able to gather additional robust evidence of their long term effects diminishes. Sadly, it means that NICE guidance not only does more harm than good in the short run, it also risks systematically undermining the evidence base for future clinical practice, with harms of unknown magnitude.

Of course, it might be regarded as unfair to say NICE has done more harm than good in terms of population health when compared to what in principle could have been done in the absence of the pressures it has undoubtedly faced. For example, what might have happened if NICE had been abandoned in 2004 or later for refusing to bend to those pressures? It seems reasonable to suppose that decision-makers would have been reluctant to approve new technologies at prices which were unaffordable at a local level and the political pressure of evident postcode prescribing and limited access to new technologies would have increased. Whether this would have led to a much needed and more effective central price negotiation mechanism is hard to say, although this did seem to be a real possibility between the publication of the Office of Fair Trading report in 2007 (Office of Fair Trading, 2007) and the election of the coalition government in 2010, which had a manifesto commitment to introduce value-based pricing (Claxton, Briggs et al., 2008). So, as well as becoming an important mechanism for imposing cost-ineffective technologies on the NHS, NICE may also have played a role in allowing policy-makers to avoid the much more politically difficult task of establishing a pricing mechanism to ensure affordable prices for the NHS.

Paradise regained?

Over time, health technology investment decisions have become increasingly complex. Manufacturers make submissions to NICE which commonly include confidential discounts to achieve NICE approval but, even when approved by NICE, they may face a second round of negotiation with NHS England if their budget impact is large. Subsequently, the same manufacturers will pay a rebate at a national level based on overall caps to the growth in total expenditure on branded pharmaceuticals. The overall transaction price for the NHS is difficult to evaluate, but the health opportunity costs falling on the local NHS remain.

Part of the explanation for this complexity may be that NICE was given two potentially conflicting tasks: i) to undertake transparent evidence-based assessment of the likely long term benefits and costs of a new technology; and ii) to make decisions about whether the technology should be approved with a funding requirement based on the price submitted by the manufacturer net of any confidential discount offered during NICE appraisal. NICE was well suited to the first task and to a large extent continues to do this well. However, the second task has placed NICE at the heart of market access and pharmaceutical pricing in the UK, which also has impacts on many other markets. Unfortunately, NICE was not provided with adequate tools and policy mechanisms to be able to do this job effectively. The only leverage NICE has is to reject a new technology, depriving *identifiable* patients of effective treatment. The only tools NICE has had at its disposal are its stated 'threshold' range and 'modifiers' and the consideration of any confidential product specific discounts offered by manufacturers.

There is a solution, and it has been available for some time. It was set out in the consultation on value-based pricing (Claxton, Sculpher and Carroll, 2011), but only now are all the required elements in place (Claxton, 2016). What is needed is a *New NICE* with one specific task in a trio of complementary decisions: i) an independent and evidence-based assessment of the additional costs and benefits of new technologies (conducted by NICE); ii) an independent (including from NICE) and evidence-based assessment of health opportunity costs; and iii) a more effective central pricing or reward mechanism which would draw on these two estimates. A centralised mechanism could be constructed in a number of ways, including a more radical de-linking of the appropriate reward of innovation from sales volumes; an option not available to a HTA body with a single stated threshold range (Woods et al., 2022). The most obvious way, however, would be to reform the current rebates paid at a national level based on caps on the growth of branded drug expenditure. Instead of crude caps on growth under the Voluntary Scheme for Branded Medicines Pricing, Access and Growth (Department of Health and Social Care, 2023), the results of NICE appraisal and an estimate of health opportunity cost could be used to establish the rebates required from manufacturers, paid at a national level which would reflect the discrepancy between the prices they wish to charge for their portfolio of products and how much the NHS can afford to pay for the benefits they provide.

De-linking NICE appraisal from *de facto* price negotiation, market access and an assessment of health opportunity costs would mean that NICE could focus on what it does best: assessing the long term costs and benefits of new drugs based on the evidence. Manufacturers can then decide if they wish to include a new drug in the national rebate agreement and pay any additional rebate that might be required as a consequence. If they do, prescribers could be fully reimbursed by the centre, incentivising early uptake of cost-effective technologies. If they do not, their product would not be rejected by NICE. It would be available but would not be reimbursed, so the full cost would fall on prescribers' budgets. NICE would no longer be placed in the politically difficult and potentially compromising position of being asked to approve or reject new drugs. The funding requirement, and the inevitable conflict with NHS England and local commissioners, would become unnecessary as all drugs included in the national rebate calculation could be fully reimbursed by the centre. A central reimbursement mechanism would remove not only reasons for geographic variation in access to new drugs but also the indirect variation in access to other care due to local funding requirements.

Such a national value-based rebate scheme would still require an assessment of how much the NHS can afford to pay for the benefits offered. This still requires some empirical assessment of health opportunity costs. However, that would no longer be the responsibility of NICE. Its stated 'threshold' range would no longer be necessary. Although a considerable body of empirical evidence about the scale of health opportunity costs in the NHS is available, there inevitably remain legitimate uncertainties. However, the important thing is that this is an empirical question that can be addressed and periodically re-estimated as more and better data become available – indeed, this may be an impetus to invest in such data. An ongoing evidence-based and accountable assessment of health opportunity costs, independent of NICE would give manufacturers the clear and predictable signal they need in making good investment decisions; aligning their incentives with what the NHS needs and how much it can afford to pay.

NICE could continue to issue guidance. But instead of being a highly redacted justification for its decision to approve or reject a new technology, it would instead set out the appraisal of evidence, supporting estimates of health effects and NHS costs. As well as informing the rebate calculations, the guidance documents could focus primarily on informing prescribers/commissioners when making choices about treatment options for particular patients, identifying limits to appropriate and reimbursed use, helping commissioners consider whether the use of a drug not included in the rebate agreement can be justified. It would enable the closer integration of NICE technology appraisal with clinical guidelines; focusing on informing clinical practice and monitoring quality of care offered at a local level.

Conclusion

Although the promise of NICE's early years became compromised, the core principles of undertaking an accountable, deliberative and evidence-based assessment of the long term costs and benefits of new technologies, drawing on all relevant evidence and supported by the best methods of analysis available, remain. So, despite the many disappointments, we still believe that early promise can be regained if policy makers address the difficult task of establishing a pharmaceutical pricing mechanism to ensure affordable prices for the NHS and de-linking NICE appraisal from market access and *de facto* price negotiation. History is long and never over. **Arise New NICE!**

References

Bovenberg, J., Penton, H. and Buyukkaramikli, N. (2021) '10 Years of End-of-Life Criteria in the United Kingdom', *Value in Health*, 24(5), pp.691–98.

Buxton, M.J., Acheson, R., Caine, N., Gibson, S. and 'O'Brien, B. (1985) *Costs and Benefits of the Heart Transplant Programmes at Harefield and Papworth Hospitals.* Department of Health and Social Security, Research Report No. 12. London: HMSO.

Chilcott, J., McCabe, C., Tappenden, P., O'Hagan, A., Cooper, N.J, Abrams, K., Claxton, K. and on behalf of the Cost-Effectiveness of Multiple Sclerosis Therapies Study Group (2003) 'Modelling the cost-effectiveness of interferon beta and glatiramer acete in the management of multiple sclerosis', *British Medical Journal* 326(7388), p.522.

Claxton, K. (2008) 'Exploring uncertainty in cost-effectiveness analysis', *Pharmacoeconomics* 26(9), pp.781–98.

Claxton, K. (2016) *Pharmaceutical Pricing: Early Access, The Cancer Drugs Fund and the Role of NICE. Policy & Research Briefing.* Available at: https://www.york.ac.uk/media/che/documents/policybriefing/Drug_prices.pdf (Accessed 20 November 2023).

Claxton, K., Briggs, A., Buxton, M., Culyer, A.J., McCabe, C., Walker, S. and Sculpher, M. (2008) 'Value based pricing for NHS drugs: an opportunity not to be missed?', *British Medical Journal* 336, pp.251–54.

Claxton, K. and Culyer, A.J. (2006) 'Wickedness or folly? The Ethics of NICE's decisions', *Journal of Medical Ethics*, 32, pp.373–77.

Claxton, K., Martin, S., Soares, M., Rice, N., Spackman, E., Hinde, S., Devlin, N., Smith, P.C. et al. (2013) *Methods for the Estimation of the NICE Cost-Effectiveness Threshold.* Centre for Health Economics (CHE) Research Paper 81. York, CHE: University of York.

Claxton, K., Martin, S., Soares, M., Rice, N., Spackman, E., Hinde, S., Devlin, N., Smith, P.C. et al. (2015) 'Methods for the estimation of the NICE cost-effectiveness threshold', *Health Technology Assessment*, 19(14).

Claxton, K., Palmer, S.J., Longworth, L., Bojke, L., Griffiths, D., McKenna, C., Soares, M.O., Spackman, E. et al. (2012) 'Informing a decision framework for when NICE should recommend the use of health technologies only in the context of an appropriately designed programme of evidence development', *Health Technology Assessment* 16(46).

Claxton, K. and Sculpher, M. (2006) 'Using value of information analysis to prioritise health research: some lessons from recent UK experience', *Pharamacoeconomics* 24(11), pp.1055–68.

Claxton, K., Sculpher, M. and Carroll, S. (2011) 'Value-based pricing for pharmaceuticals: its role, specification and prospects in a newly devolved NHS'. (CHE Research Paper, No. 60). Available at: https://www.york.ac.uk/media/che/documents/papers/researchpapers/CHERP60_value_based_pricing_for_pharmaceuticals.pdf (Accessed 20 November 2023).

Claxton, K., Sculpher, M. and Drummond, M.F. (2002) 'A rational framework for decision making by the National Institute for Clinical Excellence', *Lancet*, 360(9334), pp.711–15.

Claxton, K., Sculpher, M., Palmer, S. and Culyer, A.J. (2015) 'Causes for concern: is NICE failing to uphold its responsibilities to all NHS patients?', *Health Economics* 24(1), pp.1–7.

Commonwealth Department of Health (1992) *Guidelines for the Pharmaceutical Industry on Preparation of Submissions to the Pharmaceutical Benefits Advisory Committee.* Canberra: APGS.

Culyer, A.J., McCabe, C., Briggs, A., Claxton, K., Buxton, M., Akehurst, R., Sculpher, M. and Brazier, J. (2007) 'Searching for a threshold, not setting one: the role of the National Institute for Health and Clinical Excellence', *Journal of Health Services Research and Policy*, 12(1), pp.56–58.

Department of Health (2017) 'Accelerated Access Collaborative for health technologies: DH Impact Assessment'. Available at: https://assets.publishing.service.gov.uk/govern ment/uploads/system/uploads/attachment_data/file/663094/Accelerated_Access_ Collaborative_-_impact_asssessment.pdf (Accessed 25 November 2023).

Department of Health and Social Care (2023) '2024 voluntary scheme for branded medi-cines pricing, access and growth: summary of the heads of agreement'. Available at: https://www.gov.uk/government/publications/2024-voluntary-scheme-for-branded-medicines-pricing-access-and-growth-summary-of-the-heads-of-agreement/2024-voluntary-scheme-for-branded-medicines-pricing-access-and-growth-summary-of-the-heads-of-agreement (Accessed 18 November 2023).

Dyer, C. (2006) 'NICE faces legal challenge over restriction on dementia drugs', *British Medical Journal*, 333, p.1085.

Ferner, R.E., Hughes, D.A. and Aaronson, J.K. (2010) 'NICE and new: appraising inno-vation', *British Medical Journal*, 340, b5493.

Gold, M.R., Siegel, J.E., Russell, L.B. and Weinstein, M.C. (1996) *Cost-Effectiveness in Health and Medicine*. New York: Oxford University Press.

Griffin, S., Claxton, K., Palmer, S. and Sculpher, M. (2011) 'Dangerous omissions: the consequences of ignoring decision uncertainty', *Health Economics*, 20(2), pp.212–24.

Gu, Y., Wang, A., Tang, H., Wang, H., Jiang, Y., Jin, C. and Wang, H. (2023) 'Compari-son of rare and common diseases in the setting of healthcare priorities: evidence of social preferences based on a systematic review', *Patient Preference and Adherence*, 17, pp.1783–97.

House of Commons Health Committee (2008) *NICE: First Report of the Health Commit-tee 2007–2008*. HC27-I. London: The Stationery Office.

Kennedy, I. (2009) *Appraising the Value of Innovation and other Benefits. A Short Study for NICE*. London: NICE.

Littlejohns, P. and Rawlins, M. (eds.) (2009) *Patients, the Public and Priorities in Health Care*. Oxford: Radcliffe.

Lomas, J., Martin, S. and Claxton, K. (2019) 'Estimating the marginal productivity of the English National Health Service from 2003 to 2012', *Value in Health*, 22(9), pp.995–1002.

Longworth, L., Bojke, L., Sculpher, M. and Tosh, J.C. (2011) 'Bridging the gap between methods research and the needs of policy makers: A review of the research priorities of the National Institute for Health and Clinical Excellence', *International Journal of Technology Assessment in Health Care*, 27(2), pp.1–8.

Longworth, L., Youn, J., Bojke, L., Palmer, S., Griffin, S., Spackman, E. and Claxton, K. (2013) 'When does NICE recommend the use of health technologies within a pro-gramme of evidence development? A systematic review of NICE guidance', *Pharma-coeconomics*, 31(2), pp.137–49.

Love-Koh, J., Cookson, R., Claxton, K., and Griffin, S. (2020) 'Estimating social vari-ation in the health effects of changes in health care expenditure', *Medical Decision Making*, 40(2), pp.170–82.

Martin, S., Lomas, J., Claxton, K. and Longo, F. (2021) 'How effective is marginal healthcare expenditure? New evidence from England for 2003/04 to 2012/13', *Applied Health Economics and Health Policy* 19, pp.885–903.

Martin, S., Claxton, K., Lomas, J. and Longo, F. (2022) 'How responsive is mortality to locally administered healthcare expenditure? Estimates for England for 2014/15', *Applied Health Economics and Health Policy*, 20, pp.557–72.

McCabe, C., Chilcott, J., Claxton, K., Tappenden, P., Cooper, C., Roberts, J., Cooper, N. and Abrams, K. (2010) 'Continuing the multiple sclerosis risk sharing scheme is unjustified', *British Medical Journal,* 340, c1786.

Miners, A.H., Garau, M., Fidan, D. and Fischer, A.J. (2005) 'Comparing estimates of cost effectiveness submitted to the National Institute for Clinical Excellence (NICE) by different organisations: retrospective study', *British Medical Journal*, 330(7482), p.65.

Ministry of Health (1994) *Ontario Guidelines for Economic Analysis of Pharmaceutical Products*. Ontario: Ministry of Health.

NICE (1999) *Appraisal of New and Existing Technologies: Interim Guidance for Manufacturers and Sponsors*. London: NICE.

NICE (2004) *Guide to the Methods of Technology Appraisal*. London: NICE.

NICE (2017) *Interim Process and Methods of the Highly Specialised Technologies Programme Updated to Reflect 2017 Changes*. London: NICE.

NICE (2022) *NICE Health Technology Evaluations: The Manual*. PMG36. London: NICE.

NICE Citizens Council (2002) *Report of the First Meeting of the NICE Citizens Council: Determining 'Clinical Need'*. London: NICE.

NICE Citizens Council (2004) *Ultra Orphan Drugs*. London: NICE.

NICE Citizens Council (2006) *Rule of Rescue*. London: NICE.

Office of Fair Trading (2007) *The Pharmaceutical Price Regulation Scheme. An OFT Market Study*. London: OFT.

Rawlins, M. and Culyer, A.J. (2004) 'National Institute for Clinical Excellence and its value judgments', *British Medical Journal,* 329, pp.224–27.

Woods, B., Fox, A., Sculpher, M. and Claxton, K. (2021) 'Estimating the shares of the value of branded pharmaceuticals accruing to manufacturers and to patients served by health systems', *Health Economics*, 30(11), pp.2649–66.

Woods, B., Lomas, J., Sculpher, M., Weatherly, H. and Claxton, K. (2022) *Achieving Dynamic Efficiency in pharmaceutical Innovation: Identifying the Optimal Share of Value, the Payments Required and Evaluating Pricing Policies*. Summary of report 065 from Policy Research Unit in Economic Evaluation of Health and Social Care Interventions. Available at: https://eepru.sites.sheffield.ac.uk/home (Accessed 25 November 2023).

3   Understanding the survival of NICE through a political science lens

David J. Hunter and Peter Littlejohns

Introduction

The NHS (National Health Service) is 75 years of age. For a third of this time the National Institute for Health and Care Excellence (NICE) has been a key part of it. Indeed, few parts of the NHS have survived for such a length of time. Since 1974, the NHS has undergone continuous reform and restructuring, resulting in only a few of the organisations making up the health service existing until today, either at national or local levels. They have survived for only a few years at best. NICE is very much an outlier and an exception. Why? And are there lessons to be derived from NICE's longevity that may be relevant for future reform initiatives and their survival?

This chapter seeks to address these questions, adopting a political science perspective to identify the key factors that appear to account for NICE's evolution and survival under successive governments. The chapter is organised around the following sections: first, some context is provided to place NICE in the wider changing health system. This is followed by a section describing why a political science approach is useful in providing insights into NICE's evolution. Several frameworks are proposed, none of which is sufficient to account for NICE's longevity. Rather, a 'pick and mix' approach is favoured, since different frameworks all possess some value and offer a range of insights and explanations. A third section explores four key topics to demonstrate how NICE was established and has adapted over its 25-year lifespan and with what impact – what strengths and weaknesses can be identified as well as examining how NICE has responded to these. A closing section looks ahead to policy developments coming onto the agenda to which NICE will need to be alert. It draws together the key factors that account for NICE's survival and success and which might merit reflection as NICE faces new challenges.

Context

Over the past 25 years, a third of its lifetime, the NHS has faced mounting challenges. In the late 1990s, it suffered lengthening waiting lists and funding cuts.

DOI: 10.4324/9781003501268-3

These were successfully tackled by the New Labour government which entered office in 1997 and injected new funds into the NHS. By the time the Coalition government came into office in 2010, the NHS was performing well and received high ratings from the public. In The Commonwealth Fund's ranking of 11 health systems and their performance, the NHS came top in all areas apart from healthy lives (Davis et al., 2014).

That was all to change with the new government and its ideological commitment to reducing public spending and shrinking the state. Under Prime Minister Cameron and Chancellor Osborne's austerity policy, public spending fell significantly from 2010 until the present time. Although the NHS was protected in relative terms, it received insufficient funding to maintain its performance and, in its 2021 report, The Commonwealth Fund ranked the UK NHS fourth (Schneider et al., 2021). It was therefore not well-placed to weather the COVID-19 pandemic which struck in early 2020. But other developments have contributed to the current crises in lack of funding, low pay, and staff shortages. In particular, the impact of Brexit on the NHS has been severe. Rather than leaving the European Union (EU) following the 2016 referendum resulting in new funding for the NHS – as was promised – the UK's departure has been entirely negative. This is especially the case in relation to staffing both in the NHS and in social care on which the NHS relies to be able to discharge patients efficiently when they no longer need hospital care. The result, post-pandemic, has been that the UK's economy is performing poorly when compared with other countries and the NHS has suffered as a consequence. The double whammy of austerity and Brexit to be followed by the pandemic created a 'perfect storm'. The upshot has been an unprecedented wave of strikes hitting the NHS. These are not solely about pay, but also about working conditions and the absence of a workforce strategy for recruiting and retaining staff. Even if such issues are eventually addressed, perhaps by a new government in 2024, they will take years to have an impact.

During this turbulent period in the NHS's history, NICE has not only survived but been able to adapt and respond to a changing political and policy environment. Established by the New Labour government as a natural development of the Evidence-Based Medicine movement, NICE quickly became a cornerstone of the new government's health policy. At the core of this policy was re-establishing NHS values of uniform quality and reduction in variation in care which had been threatened by Thatcherite quasi-market experiments during the 1980s and early 1990s.

Over its lifespan, NICE was subject to three changes of government – New Labour (1997–2010), Coalition (Conservatives and Liberal Democrats, 2010–2015), and Conservative (2015 to present) and 13 Secretaries of State for Health (five of whom have held office in the four years since 2019). While several health and other quangos were created and abolished over this period, often the result of 'quango culls' intended to reduce bureaucracy and spending, NICE not only survived intact but extended its remit. Which is not to say all has been plain sailing. Although its existence was never seriously threatened, there were times under the Coalition government when NICE went through a difficult period as it came under scrutiny and had to manage budget cuts in keeping with the government's wish to control public spending.

Why NICE was able not only to survive but also to extend its remit remains something of a puzzle in public policy. The Institute is an exception given that many quangos simply come and go or, if they remain, they rarely grow and develop or enjoy the high-profile NICE has had under successive governments. To explore such issues and identify those factors accounting for NICE's survival, we adopt a political science approach.

Why a political science approach?

The relevance and value of adopting a political science lens through which to study any aspect of health policy merits attention (Hunter, 2016). The role of politics in understanding complex, messy health systems is central and is why political science with its insights and frameworks is uniquely well-placed to explore and account for their inner workings (Clavier and de Leeuw, 2013). Largely ignored until recently in this context, the discipline has much to offer those seeking a deeper understanding of health systems, how they operate and adapt, and what needs to occur if they are to undergo effective and sustainable transformation. Politics is at the heart of all that happens, or fails to happen, in public policy and in complex systems, like health, with their multiple levels of decision-making and myriad groups of stakeholders conducting power plays to advance and achieve their ends (Marmor and Klein, 2012; Hunter, 2015).

Frameworks

There are numerous political science theories and frameworks that might be adopted to illustrate and understand NICE's journey and survival. What follows is not an exhaustive listing of frameworks but a quick canter through some of those which may offer the most value in addressing the concerns of this chapter and the topics selected for closer study in the next section.

First, there is the TAPIC governance framework developed by the European Observatory on Health Systems and Policies and adopted by WHO. TAPIC comprises five domains: Transparency, Accountability, Participation, Integrity, and Capacity (Greer et al., 2019). Relevant to the last of these domains is the notion of policy capacity.

A policy capacity typology has been devised, comprising skills and competences organised into three types – analytical, operational, political. Each of these operates at three distinct levels when it comes to resources and capabilities – individual, organisational and systemic (Wu, Ramesh and Howlett, 2015).

From the nine types of policy capacity generated, it is hypothesised that high levels of capacity are linked to better policy outputs and outcomes, while capacity deficits are viewed as major causes of policy failure and suboptimal outcomes. A key feature of the conceptual framework advanced by Wu and colleagues is that it covers all policy processes, including agenda-setting, formulation, decision-making, implementation and evaluation. Importantly, adequate capacity in carrying out one task does not guarantee the effective performance of other functions. Studying how NICE has performed in respect of all these processes, and with what degree of success, is the subject of the next section on topics.

Another useful, and much-used, framework is the multiple streams approach comprising three Ps – Problem, Policy, Political (Kingdon, 1997). When these three streams converge, as occurred when NICE was announced in 1997, a 'policy window' opens, enabling change to take place. NICE was seen as the optimal solution to the rationing problem that was vexing politicians at the time and dragging them into decisions about who should, and who should not, receive treatment. An independent and respected agency whose business was informed by sound evidence and research enabled the rationing issue to be taken out of politics. While it did not resolve all the difficult political issues which swirled around rationing decisions, it took the heat out of most of them and, for the most part, kept politicians at a distance.

Another relevant framework focuses on the role of administrative politics which revolves around the discretionary decisions of administrative agencies like NICE. The behaviour of any agency hinges upon several complex factors including the nature of its task, its formal powers, and its environment (Self, 1977). A complex adaptive systems framework might be included here since one of NICE's success factors lies in its ability to adapt and learn while remaining alert and attentive to the changing policy environment. Context is all-important and over NICE's 25-year history this has changed a great deal. NICE can be viewed as occupying an advocacy coalition comprising pressure groups, politicians, policy advisers, academics, and other experts as well as professionals, civil servants, and providers, all of whom endorsed a particular set of ideas and beliefs about policy in a particular policy subsystem (Baggott, 2007).

Principal-Agent Analysis (PAA) is a well established approach to exploring the relationships between governments and the bodies that they create to support them. Waterman and Meier have broadened the concept by creating a dynamic framework based on their thesis that goal conflict and information asymmetry (the mainstays of principal-agent theory) are not necessarily constant (Waterman and Meier, 1998). This methodology has been applied in one of the very few empirical studies exploring the longevity of NICE (Littlejohns et al., 2017). Applying a modified form of PAA, it was possible to map NICE and other NHS quality-related organisations onto the framework and their transience between the different states, as described by Waterman and Meier, could be assessed over time.

Finally, there is the receptive contexts for change framework comprising several factors viewed as instrumental in enabling successful change to occur (Pettigrew, Ferlie and McKee, 1992). Five key factors are of particular relevance: Environmental pressure; Quality and coherence of policy; Key people leading change; Supportive organisational culture; and Managerial-health profession relations.

Rather than settle upon any one of the above frameworks a preferable approach is to adopt a 'pick and mix' approach, or what has been termed a 'multiple lens' approach (Sabatier, 1999). This is because elements of all these frameworks can contribute to, and enrich, our understanding of NICE and its journey over a quarter of a century.

Topics

It is not possible in this chapter to do justice to every aspect of NICE and its evolution over a lengthy period of intense health policy activity and reform. Therefore, a selective approach has been adopted, highlighting those topics which appear to have been most instrumental in NICE's development, survival, and impact. A research project assessing the reasons for NICE's longevity identified ten themes: socio-political environment; governance and accountability; external relationships; clarity of purpose; organisational reputation; leadership and management; organisational stability; resources; organisational methods; and organisational performance (Littlejohns et al., 2017). For our analysis we have chosen four topics: structure and governance, e.g. moving from being a Special Health Authority to a Non-Departmental Public Body; the move to whole systems working, embracing not only clinical care but also public health and, more recently, social care; implementation and take-up of guidance; and enablers for survival in a changing policy and political context.

In exploring each of these topics, a critical assessment of their respective strengths and weaknesses is provided – what has, and what has not, worked – drawing on the political science frameworks described in the previous section.

Structure and governance

A central part of NICE's success and endurance has been its structure and governance, in particular an ability to keep its distance from government, thereby retaining its independence and the high regard in which it was held by key stakeholders. These included Big Pharma, which might be expected to be opposed to a body like NICE. In practice, Big Pharma took the view that while some of NICE's decisions might not be in its favour, many others would meet its approval (Timmins, Rawlins and Appleby, 2016).

Getting the balance right between being sufficiently close to government to remain on top of policy developments on the one hand and, on the other hand, being sufficiently independent in order not to allow political factors to cloud its judgement or influence its decisions on which interventions to support required sensitive antennae and continuous vigilance, especially on the part of the Chair and Chief Executive, supported by the Board.

It is important to stress that securing NICE's respected position, both in the UK and internationally, required a combination of structural and cultural factors, including leadership skills and ensuring close relationships were in place with Ministers, senior civil servants, the medical profession, and others. Another key factor in NICE's favour was the stability at the top of the organisation. Its first Chair, Mike Rawlins, was in post from the start until 2013, to be replaced by David Haslam, a non-executive director, who stood down in 2020. The current Chair is Sharmila Nebhrajani, who came into post new to NICE. Its first Chief Executive, Andrew Dillon, was in post until 2016 to be replaced by his deputy, Gillian Leng, who had been at NICE since 2004 (as head of guidelines). She stood down for personal reasons in 2021. NICE's founding Clinical and Public Health Director, Peter Littlejohns, was in post from its inception until 2012. Finally, Andrea Sutcliffe, Director of Finance and Deputy CEO, was in post from 2000 to 2007.

Such factors proved to be highly important although they are often ignored or overlooked in a system where churn and turnover among leaders and others at the top of organisations is seen as inevitable and part of the culture. NICE showed there was another way to succeed.

Indeed, it was testimony to the high regard in which NICE was held by governments of all hues that the Conservative-dominated Coalition government changed its status from being a special health authority to a non-departmental public body. The move made NICE less subject to ministerial direction by putting it onto a new and more independent legal footing. No longer could ministers easily abolish NICE or radically change its remit on a whim. Being accorded a formal degree of independence provided distance from politicians and, in the process, enhanced NHS's position and esteem among key players both in the UK and globally.

Revisiting our political science frameworks, NICE's remarkably painless birth was made possible by the coming together of Kingdon's multiple streams – problem, policy, politics. There was a clear problem confronting government – rationing being viewed as a 'burning platform' or 'policy window' that urgently needed attention – and the policy solution to it was one that appealed to the key stakeholders despite some concerns and misgivings. These became apparent especially among some clinicians who worried that their freedom to decide which treatments to prescribe might be eroded, and in Big Pharma anxious about disinvestment in treatments viewed by NICE as not being cost-effective. But even among those potentially threatened by NICE, or uneasy about the impact of its decisions, there was at the same time a belief that it offered opportunities and something positive.

Finally, in terms of the politics, the motivation and opportunity to do something existed with the arrival of a new government in 1997 and the 'crisis' in the NHS top among its priorities. NICE had an unexpected 'product champion' and ally in the shape of the Secretary of State for Health at the time, Frank Dobson. His engagement in the setting up of NICE, including being the inspiration behind its name (although a number of politicians of both colours have claimed paternity for the birth of the 'concept of a NICE'), was invaluable in smoothing the passage to its creation. It was Dobson's attempt to limit the prescription of Viagra to patients with specific medical conditions being deemed unlawful that reinforced his drive for an independent organisation to make these decisions based on legally acceptable criteria (see further Chapter 9).

NICE also benefitted from the existence of a receptive context for change. While the evidence was available, the process of assembling and applying it had largely to be invented from scratch (Timmins, Rawlins and Appleby, 2016). However both NICE's main guidance programmes – Health Technology and Clinical Guidelines – were able to build on an emerging research appreciation of how to get evidence into practice. As discussed in Chapter 1, there were already regional health technology appraisal groups in place which were then subsumed into one national one. Indeed, it was variation in their decision-making that was one of the stimuli for its genesis. Also, a major EU-funded project had determined how clinical guidelines should be developed (Cluzeau et al., 2003). This was then enacted by NICE to form the basis of its clinical guidelines and, subsequently, its public health guidelines programme.

As the appraisal guidance started to be developed and some decisions were 'No', the government at the time was concerned that the methods employed by NICE should be understood and accepted by patients and the public. In response, NICE created the Citizens Council (Littlejohns and Rawlins, 2009). However, there was no interference from the government and time and space were allowed for NICE's governance and operating procedures to be devised and put in place. The key people leading change in NICE's early days were therefore critical to its success and set the course it pursued for the next 25 years.

However, as noted in Chapter 1, the convergence of the three Ps did undergo a significant challenge in 2010 with the introduction of the Cancer Drugs Fund, a move on the part of the Coalition government which, however unintentionally, undermined NICE's primary purpose. The Fund was by way of delivering on Prime Minister David Cameron's promise to make available to cancer patients expensive drugs rejected by NICE for use in the NHS because of their high cost and limited effectiveness. These drugs can offer relief and an improved quality of care but only over a period of a few months. As a political move it proved popular, but was not without controversy. Some patient groups believed that the pharmaceutical companies manufacturing these expensive drugs were over-charging for them as a result of the Cancer Drugs Fund having been introduced, while others complained of being the victims of discrimination and queried why cancer should be accorded special treatment over other life-threatening conditions (Littlejohns et al., 2016). Also, the regional way in which the fund was set up led to variation in the availability of cancer drugs.

In the end, the Fund exceeded its budget limit and the responsibility for its future management was taken over by NHS England and NICE. In practice it became part of what NICE had previously called its 'only in research' category. Conditional approval was given on the basis that data would be collected so cost-effectiveness could be assessed at a later date. What had appeared to be a consensus across political parties concerning NICE and its remit began to look problematic. Indeed, the Fund did undermine NICE in overturning its recommendations and acting as a parallel rationing body (Rid et al., 2015). Many economists, including Carl Klaxton, considered the Fund to have been a waste of money as well as undermining NICE. He was reported in the *Observer* newspaper stating: 'quite frankly, this has been an appalling, unfair use of NHS resources' (McKie, 2015). It may have helped that Simon Stevens, NHS CEO, had been health advisor to Number 10 and also to Frank Dobson when NICE was established in 1999. However, Stevens conceded in the NHS England's *NHS Five Year Forward View* strategy document that changes in NICE's assessment and prioritisation processes might be necessary to reflect concerns and pressures on health care, including greater awareness of patient views and expectations (NHS Executive, 2014). Such concerns reflect the importance of a policy capacity typology noted in the previous section and, in particular, having the requisite resources and capabilities in place.

The Cancer Drugs Fund was not the only occasion when politics intruded into NICE's decisions. Earlier, the New Labour Secretary of State for Health, Patricia Hewitt, encouraged Primary Care Trusts to allow the cancer drug Herceptin to be made available to all those who might benefit from it before NICE had reached a decision on it. In the end, NICE approved the drug and open political dissent was not seen again.

What these two examples show is that while the issue of rationing seemed largely resolved with the advent of NICE, nothing can be taken for granted and political forces will always intrude if individual ministers feel so inclined. If Kingdon's multiple streams are not all converging then the potential for disruption is always a risk. Nothing is permanent and many of the policy problems that might have been thought to have been resolved have a tendency to resurface.

Move to whole systems working

A further major change to NICE, authorised by the Coalition government, concerned extending its remit to include social care. This followed an earlier move in April 2005 for NICE to assume responsibility for public health from another body, the Health Development Agency (HDA), when, keeping the NICE acronym, it had been renamed the National Institute for Health and Clinical Excellence (see Chapter 7). In some ways, taking on social care was a logical next step, although it did pose a challenge to NICE's operating model and evidence-gathering processes. The inclusion of social care in its remit also necessitated another name change with the 'C' word becoming 'Care'.

The marriage of clinical care and public health was not immediately seen as an obvious one given NICE's origins and there were concerns that public health would remain in the shadows of its clinical guidelines work. Thanks to the Centre for Public Health Excellence (CPHE) located within NICE under Mike Kelly's leadership following his move from the HDA, the concerns were unfounded while the CPHE remained in existence. As part of a major internal reorganisation in 2013 the Centre was closed, and Kelly left NICE. Public health was merged with social care (see p. 122) to form a new division of health and social care. There were many critics of the changes, including among the non-executive directors, but they did not manage to succeed in preventing them from being implemented. Since then, public health has not recovered its previous high profile within NICE or, arguably, outside it, as responsibility for public health was given to local government following the Health and Social Care Act 2012 reforms. The reasons for this are hard to pinpoint but the replacement of a senior member of the executive team who was well respected within the public health community with a middle-ranking manager with no public profile may have been a factor.

The arrival of social care in 2013 raised other concerns within NICE since it was not equipped to handle this sector and the different challenges it posed to the Institute's working practices. In particular, the nature of, and what constitutes, evidence in social care is different from that deemed appropriate or acceptable in clinical care. NICE had to equip itself with the necessary expertise without diluting its existing strengths. Moreover, its NHS-facing role had to be adapted so that it faced a different system, namely, local government which, in England, is responsible for public health and social care. Once again, the policy capacity typology was an issue in order to ensure that NICE remained fit for purpose. As noted in the previous section, adequate capacity in the clinical sphere did not axiomatically guarantee effectiveness in other spheres.

It is by no means certain if that challenge has been successfully met. The view within NICE was that it had much to offer social care given its experience in constructing guidelines that included cost-effectiveness assessments. It was thought that the rigour of its systems and processes combined with its health economic skills would be brought to bear on social care. However, not all those involved in generating evidence in social care agreed or thought that NICE had all the answers and that all was required was for local government to adopt the new guidance. A problem was that, even if there was a desire to follow the guidance, local authorities did not have the funds to implement it given the public spending cuts arising from austerity which have hit local government particularly hard from 2010 until the present.

Although the inclusion of public health, and to a greater extent social care, presented NICE with major challenges, the fact that the Institute now embraces the whole care pathway from prevention through to social care and care in the community is both a strength and opportunity especially with the creation of 42 Integrated Care Systems across England set out in the Health and Care Act 2022. Whole systems thinking, with an emphasis on population health and integrated care, means that NICE is well-positioned to respond to such developments within its extended remit. Indeed, the Institute is better placed for such a task than much of the NHS. Whether it will be able to take full advantage of these policy developments and opportunities is as yet unclear.

Implementation and take-up of guidance

Regardless of the methodological challenges it faces, NICE's success is dependent on how far its guidance is both accepted and acted upon. Otherwise, it exists as a producer of useful evidence and advice but without having real traction on the system of decision-making at a local level. Local health organisations are expected to adopt NICE technology appraisals within three months of publication. Other NICE guidance needs to be taken into consideration when decision-makers determine local priorities and make resource allocation decisions, although they may also decide to act differently in meeting health care needs. NICE guidance is not binding on local practitioners whose knowledge and skills remain important, but they would need to have good reasons for not following the guidance.

At a time when budgets are being tightly squeezed and there are severe constraints on how far NICE's guidance to invest in new treatments will be adhered to, advice on disinvestment becomes more critical. At the outset, NICE's guidance on what to invest in, and conversely what to disinvest in, was both welcome and acted upon by those making such decisions in the NHS. It was also a period of sound investment in the NHS, which ended in 2010. It can therefore no longer be assumed that this will remain the case when the NHS, public health and social care are under extreme financial pressure as they have been over the past 13 years. When it comes to disinvestment decisions, NICE may have a more important role in the financial climate in which it finds itself. Indeed, one of the recommendations from a study commissioned by NICE into its practices was the need 'to develop an active policy on disinvestment by the NHS in products which do not offer value for money' (Kennedy, 2009: 7). While there had always been 'disinvestment' advice to the NHS, NICE made this aspect of its work more accessible.

Implementing NICE guidance has always been an area of weakness. As its first chief executive, Andrew Dillon, stated: 'there is little point in us developing guidance if no one puts it into practice' (Dillon, 2007). To tackle the issue, and thereby strengthening its capacity, NICE established a dedicated team to support local NHS organisations. A full complement of implementation support tools was also available and accompanied each piece of guidance issued. A series of commissioning guides was also produced to provide information on where disinvestment might be possible and where spending might be reduced on treatments that do not improve care or represent value for money. But it is well-known that the mere provision of information and evidence is no guarantee of subsequent action. It is one factor among many in the context of policy change; and probably not the most important. Clinician attitudes, culture, custom and practice, financial stability etc. are all probably more significant influences on decision-making. Overcoming the barriers to changing practice is also a matter of concern to NICE since its work ultimately has minimal value unless these issues are understood and confronted.

Related to the issue of implementation is the volume of guidance, which carries a cost, and how far it is up-to-date and fit for purpose given the rapid pace of change in medicine. There were complaints that much of the early guidance was out-of-date and that NICE had been slow to revise its practices and methods in order to speed up the updating process (MacSweeney et al., 2022). Having outdated guidance made it easier for critics to dismiss and ignore it. Once again, the issue of policy capacity became one of importance for NICE's functioning and reputation.

Enablers for survival in a changing policy and political context

In many ways this topic underpins the others because it draws attention to the administrative politics governing NICE's operating culture. Thanks to the initial senior team and their respected career histories, experiences and skill sets, supported by a diverse board, NICE developed strong relationships inside government as well as with key stakeholders in the NHS, academia, patient groups and Big Pharma. Investing in, and maintaining these was critical to establish NICE's place in the NHS community and to earn its respect and credibility. NICE's stability in terms of its senior staff and overall longevity contributed greatly to the development of such relationships.

Overall, NICE met the criteria set out under the TAPIC framework described in an earlier sub-section. From the outset, efforts were made to ensure that NICE's business was conducted in public and in various locations around

England but also with attention paid to links with Wales, Scotland and Northern Ireland. In an effort to be open and transparent and to engage with people and issues in the NHS and beyond, Board meetings were conducted in various locations. The format was for the Board to meet in private in the mornings, usually inviting local health managers and others to share their local issues, and then for the Board to meet in public after lunch, inviting attendees to ask questions concerning any aspect of NICE's work programme. The lunches were open to all attending the Board meetings and were an opportunity for members of the public and local NHS staff to meet with, and talk directly to, senior NICE staff. Indeed, when there was a Multiple Sclerosis Society demonstration outside the hospital where the Board meeting was taking place against NICE's decision on Beta Interferon, the demonstrators were invited to join the lunch and to attend the Board meeting.

As part of its outreach philosophy and in an effort to avoid being seen as London-centric, NICE established an office in Manchester. Although its headquarters remained in London, much of the work on guidelines and assessments was done from the Manchester office which employed over 300 staff. Having a base in the North of England contributed to NICE's connectivity to the NHS, to a wider range of academics, and the broader general public across the country.

The Institute saw its legitimacy and credibility arising from being connected to the NHS at all levels, and not just upwards to government. Outreach was seen to be a vitally important part of its mission. One of the key features of NICE's success was its ability to be at the interface between the emerging initiatives developed by the NHS to create the evidence on which it could base its decisions, and the new managerial monitoring systems that the New Labour government had put in place to assess progress against its aspirations. While the NHS R&D initiative was continuing to evolve, and was subsequently formalized into the National Institute for Health Research, NICE provided that link between the science and what was needed in practice.

Participation was also a key priority for NICE. The often used maxim 'if you are likely to be affected by the decision you have a right to be part of the decision' was rigorously adhered to. NICE engaged a wide range of experts from the NHS, academia and elsewhere to be members of its various committees producing the appraisal guidance, and created a series of national collaborating centres to generate clinical guidelines. On occasion, these could give rise to conflicts of interest and concerns over bias such as in the case of the back pain guideline in 2009 (Rawlins and Littlejohns, 2009). In this case the President of the British Pain Society, Paul Watson, was forced to resign after a campaign from members who were unhappy with the NICE guidelines on the management of low back pain which he helped develop. NICE's Chair and the Institute's clinical and public health director in a letter to the *British Medical Journal* called the move 'shameful' and 'professional victimisation of the worst kind' (Rawlins and Littlejohns, 2009). But the incident was the exception and overall the NICE approach was viewed as a strength.

The final two components of the TAPIC framework – Integrity and Capacity – were also features of NICE's operating style. It set great store by its commitment to integrity. It did not get everything right but it did commit to being a listening organisation and, while it generally stood by its judgements, it was not so inflexible that it would not review decisions when it seemed prudent to do so. Finally, in terms of capacity, NICE invested heavily in ensuring a skilled and committed workforce. Whether this applied equally across the three domains of clinical care, public health and social care, is perhaps open to argument and may be something to consider as NICE goes forward.

Conclusion

In this chapter we have sought to demonstrate how insights from political science can usefully illuminate NICE's evolution and survival during its first 25 years. Its longevity has in many ways been remarkable in a context which, over the period, has become increasingly turbulent and uncertain with successive governments, especially since 2010, displaying greater hostility to public bodies as a result of being wedded to an ideology centred on small government and shrinking the state. Mounting churn within government affecting departments and ministerial appointments has reinforced a chronic short-termism in policy-making.

Notwithstanding such a difficult and highly charged political environment, NICE has displayed a resilience, and an ability to navigate a path, that has enabled it to retain its independence and, for the most part, to maintain its founding values and ethos. Whether that legacy can survive the next few, let alone 25, years, and what lessons the past can offer for the future are topics explored in the final chapter of this book.

References

Baggott, R. (2007) *Understanding Health Policy*. Bristol: Policy Press.

Clavier, C. and de Leeuw, E. (2013) 'Framing public policy in health promotion: ubiquitous, yet elusive', in Clavier, C. and de Leeuw, E. (eds) *Health Promotion and the Policy Proc*ess. Oxford: Oxford University Press, pp.1–22.

Cluzeau, F., Burgers, J., Brouwers, M., Grol, R., Mäkelä, M., Littlejohns, P., Grimshaw, J. and Hunt C. (2003) 'Development and validation of an international appraisal instrument for assessing the quality of clinical practice guidelines: the AGREE project', *Quality and Safety in Health Care*, 12, pp.18–23.

Davis, K., Stremikis, K., Squires, D. and Schoen, C. (2014) *Mirror, Mirror on the Wall, 2014 Update: How the US Health Care System Compares Internationally*. New York: The Commonwealth Fund.

Dillon A. (2007) 'Using evidence to inform practice: Lessons from NICE', Consilium Scientific. 2024. Available at: https://www.consilium-scientific.org/all-speakers/103-transcript/373-using-evidence-to-inform-practice-lessons-from-nice (Accessed 14 April 2024).

Greer, S.L., Vasev, N., Jarman, H., Wismar, M. and Figueras, J. (2019) 'It's the governance, stupid! TAPIC: a governance framework to strengthen decision making and implementation', Health Systems and Policy Analysis, Policy Brief 33, European Observatory on Health Systems and Policies. Copenhagen: WHO.

Hunter, D.J. (2015) 'Role of politics in understanding complex, messy health systems: an essay', *British Medical Journal* 350:h1214.

Hunter, D.J. (2016) *The Health Debate*. 2nd edn. Bristol: Policy Press.

Kennedy, I. (2009) *Appraising the Value of Innovation and Other Benefits. A Short Study for NICE*. London: NICE.

Kingdon, J. (1997) *Agendas, Alternatives and Public Policies*. 2nd edition. New York: Harper Collins.

Littlejohns, P. and Rawlins, M. (eds) (2009) *Patients, the Public and Priorities in Health Care*. Oxford: Radcliffe.

Littlejohns, P., Knight, A., Littlejohns, A., Poole, T.-L. and Kieslich, K. (2017) 'Setting standards and monitoring quality in the NHS 1999–2013: a classic case of goal conflict', *International Journal of Health Planning and Management*, 32(2), pp.e185-e205.

Littlejohns, P., Weale, A., Kieslich, K., Wilson, J., Rumbold, B., Max C. and Rid, A. (2016) 'Challenges for the new Cancer Drugs Fund', *Lancet Oncology*, 17(4), pp.416–18.

MacSweeney, S., Subramanian, G., Podlase, A. and Auer, D. (2022) 'Urgent need to update NICE guidelines on imaging for transient ischaemic attack', *The Lancet*, 400(10349), p.357.

Marmor, T. and Klein, R. (2012) *Politics, Health and Health Care: Selected Essays*. New Haven: Yale University Press.

McKie, R. (2015) 'David Cameron's flagship Cancer Drugs Fund "is a waste of NHS cash"', *The Observer* (10 January). Available at: https://www.theguardian.com/politics/2015/jan/10/cancer-drugs-fund-waste-of-nhs-cash-david-cameron (Accessed 5 April 2023).

NHS Executive (2014) *Five Year Forward View*. London: NHS Executive.

Pettigrew, A., Ferlie, E. and McKee, L. (1992) *Shaping Strategic Change*. London: Sage Publications.

Rawlins, M. and Littlejohns, P. (2009) 'NICE outraged by ousting of pain society president', *British Medical Journal*, 339:b3028.

Rid, A., Littlejohns, P., Wilson, J., Rumbold, B., Kieslich, K. and Weale, A. (2015) 'The importance of being NICE', *Journal of the Royal Society of Medicine*, 108(10), pp.385–89.

Sabatier, P.A. (1999) 'The need for better theories', in Sabatier P.A. (ed) *Theories of the Policy Process*. Oxford: Westview Press, p.3–20.

Schneider, E.C., Shah, A., Doty, M.M., Tikkanen, R., Fields, K. and Williams II, R.D. (2021) *Mirror, Mirror 2021: Reflecting Poorly*. Online. Available at: https://www.commonwealthfund.org/publications/fund-reports/2021/aug/mirror-mirror-2021-reflecting-poorly (Accessed 7 April 2023).

Self, P. (1977) *Administrative Theories and Politics*. 2nd edn. London: Allen & Unwin.

Timmins, N., Rawlins, M. and Appleby, J. (2016) *A Terrible Beauty: A Short History of NICE*. Thailand: Health Intervention and Technology Assessment Programme.

Waterman, R.W. and Meier, K.J. (1998) 'Principal-agent models: An expansion?', *Journal of Public Administration Research and Theory*, 8(2), pp.173–202.

Wu, X., Ramesh, M. and Howlett, M. (2015) 'Policy capacity: A conceptual framework for understanding policy competences and capabilities', *Policy and Society*, 34(3–4), pp.165–71.

4 NICE's paradigm of public practical reasoning

Albert Weale

Introduction

For those who study the role of ideas in the policy process, NICE offers a fascinating case-study of public practical reasoning. During the first 20 years or so of its existence – the period that we might think of as the 'classical' phase of its thinking – NICE's decision-making rested on an articulated substantive paradigm of public decision-making, in which the fundamental principle was that of prioritising cost-effective interventions within health services assuming a given level of expenditure determined by government. The key elements of this paradigm included such concepts as the incremental cost-effectiveness ratio, quality-adjusted life-years (QALYs) and opportunity costs. These concepts were embedded in practices of health technology appraisal that were impressive in themselves and were highly regarded internationally. They were also said to provide the public justification for the decisions on particular technologies that NICE made. They were rationalised by reference to the idea of 'social value judgements', set out with admirable clarity in the document called *Social Value Judgements* (NICE, 2008). They also reflected long-standing theoretical thinking, particularly in welfare economics and the economics of social policy, about the role of the government in promoting health and social welfare.

I conjecture that part of the success of NICE – and, judging by the expansion of its functions over time, NICE has been a success – was due to its being able to take the vague rhetoric used by politicians and commentators of 'getting the best value for money' from the public services and producing an operational model that could claim to embody that ambition. Since, behind the operational model was some sophisticated economic thinking, 'common sense' could be reconstructed as economic rigour. Moreover, any system of collective health coverage – whether it be private insurance, social insurance or tax-based funding – needs to be able to determine what is a 'good buy' that merits coverage in the collective plan as against interventions that should be left to a private contractual relationship between patient and supplier. For example, if the collective scheme does not cover homeopathy, there need be

DOI: 10.4324/9781003501268-4

nothing to stop patients obtaining the intervention through private practice: it is simply not part of the health care package that is collectively supplied through government funding or regulation. Moreover, since good medicine is not coextensive with expensive medicine, any parsimony that NICE imposed on NHS services could be counted as a medical benefit in itself. In this context, NICE's 'do not do' recommendations were an important component of its work. The paradigm that NICE employed was thus simultaneously a tool of public administration and the expression of a policy culture that gave high value to proven clinical effectiveness on a sound financial basis.

Paradigms come with implications, however. In particular, as NICE developed and applied its paradigm to a number of specific cases and addressed a number of morally complex issues – including end of life interventions, a clash with professional judgements about good clinical practice, and access to innovative therapies – its decisions were at odds with the application of a cost-benefit paradigm. Critics of NICE were quick to allege that these departures showed weakness of will, muddled thinking or deference to lobbying. Another interpretation, however, is that there can be overreach in applying one single paradigm to complex questions of priority-setting in a mechanistic way. Whilst it is laudable to apply rigour in a good cause, there is always the question as to whether the rigour leads to such anomalies that one doubts whether the cause itself is quite as unambiguously good as one initially supposes. That is the interpretation to be explored in this chapter. In particular, I shall suggest that the anomalies that arose in the application of the NICE classical paradigm were expressions of the latent tensions and conflicts in the thinking behind that paradigm.

My approach will be first, in Section 2, to set out the key elements of NICE's classical paradigm and its account of social value judgements. Section 3 locates that paradigm in a brief intellectual history of the evolution of twentieth-century welfare economics from nineteenth-century utilitarianism. Section 4 explores the problems associated with the ethics of opportunity costs, given that a concern with opportunity costs has been central to the NICE approach. Section 5 shows how the tensions and conflicts implicit in the classical paradigm played out NICE's decision-making in particular appraisals. Section 6 concludes by asking how significant is the shift in 2020 from the language of social value judgements to the language of principles.

The classical paradigm

From its inception until 2020, when it formally issued new principles for the guidance of its guidance and standards (NICE, 2020), NICE worked on the basis of a particular, well-articulated paradigm of decision-making. It was set out in *Social Value Judgements* (NICE, 2008) and I shall refer to it as the 'classical paradigm'. That paradigm is generally well known and is laid out by others in this volume. However, for the sake of convenience, I detail its principal features here.

The classical paradigm is a calculus of decision-making. That is to say, it contains core concepts linked by chains of reasoning to draw practical conclusions as to what should be done. Within this calculus, the key concepts are: the QALY; the incremental cost-effectiveness ratio; and the threshold.

The QALY is the measure of benefit preferred by NICE (NICE, 2008: 17). It combines information both on increases in life-expectancy following an intervention and on improvement in the quality of life secured by that intervention. The latter is usually captured using the EQ-5D measure of quality of life, across five dimensions: mobility, capacity for self-care, ability to carry out one's usual activities, pain or discomfort, and anxiety and depression. As is well known, the QALY measure combines the value of added years and quality of life by discounting the value of any added years by an estimate of the associated quality of life. For example, an added year of life in great pain might be worth only half of an added year of life with no pain. *Social Value Judgements* (NICE, 2008: 17) justified the use of QALYs by saying that it was important to capture the value of health interventions that improved the quality of life as well as interventions that extended life. So, to use an example not cited by NICE, the development of anti-hypertensive drugs since the early formulations of the 1950s have largely been aimed at reducing adverse side-effects like sweating or erectile dysfunction. The use of the QALY measure enables assessments to capture the value of such improvements.

An additional important reason for using the QALY measure offered by *Social Value Judgements* (NICE, 2008: 17) is that it enables comparison across different interventions for different conditions. What this means is that by using QALYs, decision-makers can compare, say, the value of coronary artery bypass grafting in preventing heart attacks to advice by GPs to patients to give up smoking (to use a well-known early example from Williams, 1985). Such comparisons then play a role in setting priorities among different interventions.

Within the NICE framework, the use of QALY comparisons is necessary for priority-setting, but not sufficient. A QALY is just a measure of value. That measure of value needs to be plugged into the decision calculus that defines when an intervention producing a QALY gain ought to be funded and when it ought not to be funded. A key stage at this point is the incremental cost-effectiveness ratio. *Social Value Judgements* defines the incremental cost-effectiveness ratio as 'the ratio of the difference in the mean costs of an intervention compared to the next best alternative (which could be no action or treatment) to the differences in the mean health outcomes' (NICE, 2008: 18). In other words, for any new intervention, subtract from its mean costs the mean costs of existing interventions. Having done that, subtract from the mean added QALYs of the new intervention the mean added QALYs of the existing intervention. Then express the cost per QALY as the ratio of the former figure over the latter.

Within the calculus, the incremental cost-effectiveness ratio will not of itself give a criterion of determining which treatments to fund and which not to fund unless there is a rule determining a cut-off point. An incremental cost-effectiveness ratio will provide information for a rank-ordering of interventions by their cost-effectiveness, but of itself does not define what is a maximum acceptable cost. Hence the need for a threshold of cost acceptability. Interventions below the threshold – that is to say interventions with a relatively low cost per QALY – will be funded, unless there are special considerations, and interventions above the threshold – that is to say interventions offering no gain above the cost of the most marginal intervention and so with a high cost per QALY – will not be funded. Both in *Social Value Judgements* and elsewhere, NICE and its Board members denied that the threshold was fixed (NICE, 2008: 18; Rawlins and Culyer, 2004: 224), but figures of between £20,000 and £30,000 per QALY were given as indicative of the point at which funding for interventions were no longer regarded as good value for the NHS. As we shall see later, precisely how the threshold operates as a decision criterion is an important point. But the general approach is clear. If an intervention comes in at below £20,000 per QALY, then generally speaking well and good. If it comes in above £20,000 to £30,000 per QALY, then some special reason needs to be given for making a positive recommendation.

As Rumbold, Weale, Rid, Wilson and Littlejohns (2017: 113–14) point out, the classical NICE system was not strictly speaking a maximising strategy in the way it operated. That is to say, it was not a strategy that secured maximum benefit for any given level of health care spending. Rather it was a satisficing strategy, in which any particular decision is regarded as 'good enough' in terms of improving efficiency in the use of healthcare resources. Thus, *Social Value Judgements* eschews the language of maximisation, pointing out that cost-effectiveness might need to be balanced by a fair allocation of resources (NICE, 2008: 18). For example, greatest health gain might be secured by concentrating resources in some regions rather than others, but fairness would require the health needs of all regions in a country to be weighed in the balance.

Nonetheless, some of those who articulated most clearly the cost-effectiveness paradigm did suggest that maximisation of benefit was its ultimate rationale. For example, in 'What Could be Nicer than NICE?', Alan Williams (2004) envisaged a process in which NICE would undertake cost-effectiveness evaluations of the full range of interventions practised by the NHS, rejecting the cost-ineffective ones and recommending the cost-effective ones. Moreover, since medical technology was constantly evolving, Williams noted that once the task had been finished, it should be started all over again. So, we can think of the Williams approach as a Forth Bridge strategy: when you have finished one round of work, you start again. To this strategy Culyer (2016) added the Bookshelf

Analogy. Imagine that you have to put books on a bookshelf, ordering them from left to right. The books are of various heights, with the higher ones standing for greater cost-effectiveness. The width of the books stands for the total cost of providing the intervention, being the average unit cost multiplied by the number patients receiving the benefit. The task is to place the books on the shelf starting from the left in height order, stopping at the point that corresponds to the total health budget, equal to the width of the books on the left side of the shelf. The height of the shortest book within the budget range gives the threshold. It follows that the summed height of all the books to the left of the total budget point is at a maximum, so that replacing a book to the left of the budget line with a book to the right of the budget line would reduce the total benefit gained from health spending. If the books are placed correctly, the equivalent of QALY maximisation is achieved.

Note that the Bookshelf Analogy crucially gives a rationale for the threshold. The threshold is derived, by construction, from the least cost-effective intervention that can be funded within the total budget, when interventions are ranked from most to least cost-effective. The use of a threshold thus simplifies the appraisal of any particular technology by answering the question: does any particular technology give benefit to the requisite degree? By requiring the technology to pass the threshold test, it enables the satisficing strategy to be applied over time and case by case. However, the use of the threshold presupposes that the crucial consideration in making a decision about a technology is the extent to which it is consistent with QALY maximisation. The rationale of the threshold test, therefore, is that, if any intervention falls short of the threshold, it is an indication that resources are not being deployed as productively they might otherwise be.

Why social value judgements?

The classical NICE paradigm is expressed in the language of 'social value judgements'. That language is not one that is drawn from common usage. To understand the idea of social value judgements, we need to locate the concept in the intellectual history of the political and economic philosophies that shaped the health economics thinking that has informed NICE's work.

In NICE's adoption of the idea of social value judgements, we are hearing the echoes of the sub-discipline of welfare economics – the study of the economic conditions under which human welfare is improved – at a particular stage of its theoretical development (Charlton and Weale, 2021). Welfare economics grew out of the utilitarianism of the nineteenth century. As a political philosophy, utilitarianism enjoined governments to maximise the value of the net benefits, or utility, associated with any course of action. In the early phases of utilitarian thought, associated with Bentham, utilitarians conceived utility as a natural property of human beings to be identified with pleasure or happiness. So the task of government was to ensure the greatest possible happiness of the greatest number. However, as a guide to government action, this principle became increasingly implausible as utilitarian thinkers themselves found it impossible to say how happiness could be measured and how one would know whether a gain in net happiness had been produced. So, in place of the idea of happiness, the task of government was seen as maximising utility seen as the 'the good' and regarded as a complex property of the world (Weale, 2020: Chapter 2). So, for example, the utilitarian in making a judgement about what was good in the world had to balance such properties as pleasure, beauty and loyalty. In place of the simple conception of utility as pleasure, there was a complex conception of utility as being made up of different heterogeneous elements.

A corresponding change took place in the development of welfare economics, the origin of which was to be found in the application of utilitarian thinking to questions of economic policy. If the utilitarians sought to maximise pleasure, early welfare economics sought to maximise that portion of human welfare that could be brought in relation to the measuring rod of money. Welfare in this sense could be seen as an objective property of the world. However, just as utilitarians developed doubts about basing judgements on pleasure as an objective property of the world, so welfare economists over time came to doubt that judgements could be based on a measure of economic welfare regarded as an objective property of the world.

This latter development was related to changes in economic thinking about welfare and choice. In particular, the idea of utility came to be identified with what individuals preferred, that is to say how they ranked alternatives according to their own subjective estimate. So, when individuals thought about social arrangements, they would come to their own balance about how the different elements of any social state were to be balanced against one another. Arrow expressed the idea with his customary clarity, having noted that according to welfare economics choice is made over 'social states':

> The most precise definition of a social state would be a complete description of the amount of each type of commodity in the hands of each individual, the amount of labor to be supplied by each individual, the amount of each productive resource invested in each type of productive activity, and the amounts of the various types of collective activity, such as municipal services, diplomacy and its continuation by other means, and the erection of statues to famous men. *It is assumed that each individual in the community has a definite ordering of all conceivable social states, in terms of their desirability to him.* (Arrow, 1963: 17, italics added)

Within this conception, there was no particular specification as to what made for social welfare in the preferences of individuals. For example, some individuals might prefer a more equal distribution of income to a less equal distribution, implying that a more equal society was better than a less equal one, whereas other individuals' judgements about what made for a better society would be the opposite. The key point was not so much the particular content of these judgements as the fact that they were derived from individuals' preferences over social alternatives. The preferences were therefore a function of the elements of the social alternatives. Hence they were thought of as a 'social welfare function'. As Harsanyi (1955: 309) put it, such a social welfare function was 'defined as an arbitrary mathematical function of economic (and other social) variables, of a form freely chosen according to one's personal ethical (or political) value judgments.' (The term 'arbitrary' in this quotation is used in the logical sense: it does not mean 'randomly compiled' but rather 'compiled of elements that can be logically substituted by other equivalent elements'.) So, in place of the simple idea of maximising that portion of welfare that could be brought in relation to the measuring rod of money, there was the complex idea that public policy should aggregate the highly variable social welfare functions of individuals to produce a grand, overall collective social welfare function.

Given that the individual social welfare functions were defined by personal or political value judgements, there was an obvious problem, however. How could one determine authoritative public policy choices given the potential multiplicity of individual social welfare judgements? One approach was to say that unanimously agreed judgements of social welfare should form the basis for public policy. However, this criterion itself raised problems. If unanimity were taken as a necessary condition of public policy choice, then conservatism would prevail. Marie Antoinette alone could have saved the royalty in France (Sen, 1970: 25). If unanimity were only sufficient, then only a vanishingly small set of decisions would be covered by the test.

In a justly famous result Arrow (1963) showed that, in the absence of unanimity, it was logically impossible to define a rule that combined individual value judgements into a collective public choice in such a way as to guarantee that the result would satisfy 'reasonable' conditions. The term 'reasonable' was used to indicate that any combined individuals' values should both be responsive to the value judgements of all the individuals in a society, whilst at the same time being coherent. Coherence meant that if alternative A were judged better than alternative B, which in turn was judged better than alternative C, then alternative A should be judged to be better than alternative C. The idea may seem abstract, but it is easy to show, for example, that majority rule, as a familiar way of making collective choices, fails to satisfy the coherence condition (Weale, 2018: Chapter 4). Arrow showed that the only way of guaranteeing coherence, in the absence of unanimity, was to make the judgements of only one individual definitive of what should be done in public policy, and so not generally responsive. In combining different views, there is a built-in conflict between being responsive to a range of individuals and in coming up with a final coherent public choice.

These developments in the logic of utilitarianism and welfare economics were exhibited in the development of the NICE classical paradigm. The obvious parallel to simple utilitarianism or simple welfare economics would be the principle that a health care system should seek to maximise QALY gain. This would be the simple conception of NICE's task. However, *Social Value Judgements* (NICE, 2008: 9) explicitly denied adopting such a utilitarian approach to its decision-making, on the grounds that it would allow the interests of the majority to outweigh those of the minority. Instead it claimed to draw on a range of values, including fairness and procedural justice. This is a more complex conception of NICE's task. In effect, NICE's rejection of simple QALY maximisation replicated the logic by which utilitarianism moved from the view that the object of government was to secure the greatest happiness for the greatest number (even if this created unhappiness for some of those affected) to the view that the task of government was to maximise the good, where the good was comprised of a number of heterogeneous elements. QALY maximisation corresponds to the simple happiness maximisation of the early utilitarianism. Similarly, QALY maximisation is the counterpart of maximising that portion of welfare that can be brought in relation to the measuring rod of money, but on the more complex conception it is not coextensive with social welfare. To the value of QALY maximisation had to be added other values, a counterpart to Harsanyi's arbitrary function in which a set of considerations incorporating diverse social values helped define what a good outcome of policy was. Table 4.1 summarises these various relationships.

That then left the problem of how different conceptions of social welfare could be combined in a satisfactory way, the problem with which Arrow had been concerned. How would one know that NICE had set the right balance between, say, QALY maximisation on the one hand and fairness to minority groups on the other? Unanimous consensus from the Citizens Council might be one way

Table 4.1 Simple and complex bases of social choice

Framework	Simple	Complex
Utilitarianism	Maximise net happiness across the population.	Maximise the good across the population.
Welfare Economics	Maximise that portion of welfare that can be brought in relation to the measuring rod of money.	Choose the best social welfare function from those that are available.
NICE (Classical)	Maximise QALY gain.	Choose according to a calculus of social values.

(see Chapter 8), but the scope of such consensus is limited. A broad congruence between the values prevalent in the UK and NICE's paradigm that has been empirically observed (see Landwehr and Klinnert, 2015) is interesting, but not in itself sufficient to overcome the problem. In the absence of complete consensus, there is no way of solving the Arrow problem of the logical impossibility of combining different views about how the component parts of social welfare were to be defined in a reasonable way. Not even NICE could overcome a logical impossibility. Instead, it has simply to be asserted, as it was by NICE, that its decisions were being made authoritatively on behalf of society. (The Hobbesian ghost in the social welfare machine, we might say.) NICE thus described itself as taking the social point of view. In practice this typically meant that it sought to take an impartial perspective, in which no particular social groups were privileged and in which all would be on an equal footing according to the principle that a QALY is a QALY is a QALY.

Despite these modifications and adaptations, there was one overarching legacy from the utilitarian and welfare economics traditions. This was the assumption that a right action or a right policy was to be judged in terms of the good that was produced as a consequence. What was right was that policy or action that was productive of the good, and the more good that was produced the more any action or policy would be justified. In this sense, for NICE the good preceded the right, to use the Rawlsian formulation (compare Rawls, 1999: 21–22). As a result, the approach made the entitlements of individuals depend on how their needs figured in some scheme of social good. That in turn raised a number of practical policy problems.

The ethics of opportunity costs

A number of reasons have been advanced to justify the classical NICE paradigm. They include the following. The paradigm substituted explicit reasoning for implicit clinical and managerial judgement, the latter being suspect precisely because it was tacit and variable rather than open and consistent. The method required manufacturers of pharmaceutical products to jump the 'fourth hurdle' of cost-effectiveness on top of the tests of effectiveness, efficacy and safety, and so prevented the NHS being burdened with costs that represented only slight marginal improvements in patient health and well-being. The use of QALYs was an improvement over previous measures of effectiveness like five-year survival rates, notably allowing the purchasing authorities to take into account quality of life improvements. The method counteracted the 'post-code lottery' by which one local health authority would supply an intervention but another, possibly one that was located just the other side of a not very wide river, would not. In all these ways, it could be argued, NICE's paradigm of decision-making could contribute to accountable practical public reasoning. With calculation at its base,

NICE nonetheless could arguably have been said to articulate through its paradigm a deliberatively reasonable set of priority judgements.

However, there is one claimed advantage of the NICE classical paradigm that some regard as being particularly important, namely in its highlighting the role of measuring opportunity costs in priority-setting decisions (Claxton and Culyer, 2006; Rumbold et al., 2017). Those who stress the significance of opportunity costs reason as follows. In a cash-limited system of health care financing, like that of the NHS, a decision to fund one set of interventions will necessarily lead to some other interventions not being funded. For example, a decision to fund an expensive anti-cancer drug that prolongs life by only a few months will lead to other interventions not being financed adequately. Where these forgone interventions are ones that would benefit the relatively vulnerable and marginalised – for example mental health outreach interventions for members of minority communities – then the ethics of opportunity cost lines up with a concern for the least advantaged. It was partly for these reasons that *Social Value Judgements* rejected the rule of rescue, emphasising that its own paradigm enabled decision-makers to 'consider the needs of present and future patients of the NHS who are anonymous and who do not necessarily have people to argue their case on their behalf' (NICE, 2008: 20). (However, for an analysis of how consistent NICE's practice has been with this rejection in respect of highly specialised technologies, see Charlton, 2022, who suggests that in these cases NICE's decision-making is consistent with the rule of rescue.)

Yet, pointing to the fact of opportunity cost alone will not lead to clear conclusions in favour of the sort of cost-effectiveness paradigm that NICE used. While it is true, for example, that cancer patients gaining an extra few months of life may impose a cost on others by their pre-empting resources, it is equally true that giving priority to those other patients would impose a cost on the cancer patients. The logic is the same as the one which Coase (1960) identified in the case of adverse spill-over effects from one economic activity to another. Coase's example, an actual legal case, was of a confectionary manufacturer whose machinery imposed noise and vibration on an adjacent medical practice so reducing the economic value of the practice. However, a restriction on the use of the machinery would reduce the value of the output of the confectionary manufacturer. The problem of cost imposition is reciprocal. The same is true with opportunity cost in a fixed health care budget system. While meeting the needs of one group of patients imposes a cost on another group of patients, meeting the needs of the second group imposes a cost on the first.

Do we have reasons for imposing the costs on one group of patients rather than another group? The proponent of QALY maximisation has a straightforward answer to this question. Deny interventions to those who, if their needs were met, would impose the greater QALY loss on others. So the answer to patients whose treatment would only prolong their lives by a few months is that the treatment ought not to be supplied because the opportunity cost, in terms of QALYs forgone, is too large. And this is seen in all interventions that fail to meet the threshold test of cost-effectiveness.

However, not only is it unclear how valid an answer this is in itself, there is an issue as to how far NICE could avail itself of such an answer. After all, one of the prime reasons given for rejecting utilitarianism as an approach in *Social Value Judgements* was to avoid the risk of making the interests of a minority subservient to the interests of a majority, and QALY maximisation may do just this. The question at this point is how far a residual utilitarianism is implicit in the NICE classical paradigm. Utilitarianism has been rejected by most modern (post-1950) social contract theorists of justice largely because it requires individuals to sacrifice their own interests for some overall social good. For example, Gauthier (1979: 10) suggested that whereas the utilitarian considers overall well-being as forming the basis of social judgement, a contractarian considers the well-being of each individual as having independent standing. Rawls (1999: 24) famously formulated the matter by noting that utilitarianism 'does not take seriously the distinction of persons'. So, whereas it makes sense for one person to make a sacrifice of some good in his or her own life in order to achieve a more highly valued good in life, it does not similarly make sense for one person, from his or her own point of view, to take a loss solely for some overall social good. Or, if it does make sense, then it does so only in the context of acts of heroism and noble self-sacrifice, not from the point of view of citizens seeking financial security in the meeting of their health care needs.

In place of the utilitarian view that individuals should be prepared to give up their own well-being, and shorten their lives, for some overall good, one approach of social contract theorists is to ask whether there is a scheme of social cooperation such that no one could reasonably reject the principles of that scheme. (For expositions of this approach, see Barry 1989: 282–92; Barry, 1995: Chapter 3; Scanlon, 1982; Scanlon, 1998, Chapter 10. Both are discussed in Weale, 2020, Chapters 9, 10 and 15.) What would an appeal to this criterion mean in the case of health care priority-setting? In particular, what might this criterion tell us as to how to allocate resources between competing claimants?

Suppose, for example, one were to say to a cancer patient requiring expensive treatment that the treatment will not be provided because to do so would impose a financial burden on the system that in turn would mean that the needs of some other patients could not be met. Could cancer patients reasonably reject the principle that a failure to meet their needs would be justified as a result of the cost of meeting the needs of others? There are grounds for saying that they could reasonably reject such a principle. It is not a principle of justice that one should lay down one's life for the greater good, even if it were a principle for saints and heroes. Moreover, the cancer patients could argue that the reason for having some form of collective coverage for high cost medical interventions is that it would be financially catastrophic for individuals to have to bear those costs on their own, whereas it may not be financially catastrophic for individuals to bear the costs of quality of life improvements out of their own pockets.

At this point, in reply, it may be argued that such patients do, however, have an obligation of fairness. As beneficiaries of a system of collectively provided health care, individuals have the duty to contribute to the maintenance of the ongoing practice and this may entail claiming only a fair share of resources. (The principle of fairness here has attracted some criticism, but something like it does seem to be embedded in the social and political cultures of societies that have collective health provision aimed at universal access.) To this claim our putative cancer patients have a clear response: however, their rejection of the denial of their claims is not an attempt to avoid the obligations of fairness, but a dispute as to what a fair system of priority-setting is.

In this context, those who suffer from conditions that require high cost interventions can also question the currency within which the threshold speci-fication is made. This need not involve raising methodological questions about the way in which QALYs are constructed, though there is certainly scope to do that since it is clear that those involved in appraisal processes are aware of the problems of QALY comparisons (Bryan, Williams and McIver, 2007). Rather, the questions would concern the extent to which a purely additive calculus of social choice was the right one. Such a calculus does not preclude a small ben-efit to a large number of people outweighing a large benefit to a small number of people, as the total costs of interventions above the threshold absorb the available budget. (With large numbers, the books on the bookshelf get thicker.) So those asked to forgo their claims on resources are not even being asked to do so for something of equivalent value to others. They might reasonably say that, although they would be prepared to accept an opportunity cost that arose from the requirement to treat other patients with needs that were just as or more serious than theirs, the same obligation does not arise from a cost aris-ing from resources being devoted to small gains in the quality of life of many people, the aggregate value of which outweighed the loss of QALYs to those with conditions that were expensive to treat.

In practice, these normative arguments are likely to be associated with some ad hoc points about the claims of opportunity cost on which the decision to reject the cancer treatment is based. Here they might say that there is no one single pot of money from which all health care has to be financed. Instead, there are sepa-rate pots across the home nations of the UK, as well as across primary care spe-cialisms like dentistry, optometry, pharmacy services and public health. There is no guarantee that these separate funds comprise a coherent QALY maximising allocation. Moreover, efficiency gains secured by not funding expensive medi-cines could easily be swallowed up by a pay increase for NHS staff, procurement inefficiencies or tax cuts made with an eye on the next election. Just as with com-mercial firms there is a large gap between profit-maximising and bankruptcy, so with health services, there is bound to be a looseness of connection between the costs involved in treating some and the costs involved in treating others.

If these arguments are correct, then patients with serious conditions, or their representatives discussing the principles of collective health coverage, could reasonably reject the QALY maximisation principle, even as one element in a decision calculus. It is not simply that other considerations should ethically be included in the decision calculus for priority-setting (though that is certainly true: for an overview that brings together the previous points and more, see Menzel, 2007). Rather it is that unqualified QALY maximisation should not be included in the social value judgements at all.

At this point it might be pointed out that NICE is committed to the principles of accountability for reasonableness, as developed by Daniels and Sabin (NICE, 2008: 10, citing Daniels and Sabin, 2002). What might be the relationship between its commitment to those principles and the argument that QALY maximisation is reasonably rejectable as a criterion of priority-setting? Accountability for reasonableness is explicated via four conditions (Daniels and Sabin, 2002: 45):

1. Publicity. The reasons for limit-setting decisions must be publicly accessible.
2. Relevance. The reasons given by a priority setter must be regarded as relevant by fair-minded people.
3. Appeals and revisions. There must be a mechanism for challenge and dispute resolution.
4. Enforcement. There must be regulation of the priority-setting process to ensure that the three previous conditions are met.

Of these four conditions, it is the relevance condition that is at issue in the present case. As Rid (2009: 14) has pointed out, the relevance condition goes beyond administratively procedural due process to set a substantive constraint on what can be chosen by a priority-setting body. So the question arises as to how one might determine what constitutes a relevant consideration and whether relevant reasons permit considerations of QALY maximisation.

The formulation of the relevance condition in *Social Value Judgements* does not offer an answer to this question. It simply says that relevance is satisfied when the grounds for reaching decisions are ones 'that fair-minded people would agree are relevant in the particular context'. Taken on its own this is clearly circular. But it would be reasonable to interpret it in the light of the discussion by Daniels and Sabin.

Daniels and Sabin (2002: 51) define fair-minded people as follows: 'Specifically, a construal of the goal will be "reasonable" only if it appeals to reasons, including values and principles, that are accepted as relevant by people who are disposed to finding ways of cooperating with each other on mutually acceptable terms.' So, the crucial test is whether QALY maximisation could plausibly be introduced into a public discussion of priority-setting by those disposed to find ways of cooperating with one another on acceptable terms.

The Daniels and Sabin formulation echoes the social contract constructions of Barry and Scanlon to which I referred earlier. However, the Daniels and Sabin formulation seems to be less constraining than the Barry/Scanlon formulations, at least as I have interpreted them, since it does not seem to preclude considerations of aggregate advantage to count as being relevant as part of the reasonable moral pluralism that accountability for reasonableness presupposes. In effect, the Daniels and Sabin formulation relativizes the notion of a 'relevant reason' to each of a range of possible ethical frameworks. For a utilitarian framework maximisation is implied; for a contractualist justice approach it is not. Thus, accountability for reasonableness does not address the question of whether it would be reasonable for someone to reject a framework in which aggregating principles were operative. (Parenthetically, it may be noted that such wide reasonable pluralism would be most naturally institutionally embodied in a system in which citizens were allowed to choose which of several social insurance schemes they were compelled to enrol rather than in a single-payer system like the NHS.)

The significance of the choice of decision frameworks can be highlighted by contrasting the NICE paradigm with the German paradigm of priority-setting used by the Institute for Quality and Efficiency in Health (IQWiG) in Germany. Central to the German paradigm, as Katharina Kieslich (2012: 377; 2020: 378–79) notes, is the test of patient-relevance. Patient-relevance is a necessary test in coming to a judgement on the priority to be given to an intervention. According to the test, a proposed pharmaceutical intervention will be relevant to patients when it produces an outcome that is clinically beneficial to those patients, for example by enabling them to live longer, reduce their symptoms or complications or improve their quality of life. However, as a necessary condition, the test of patient-relevance also has an exclusionary aspect. If patient-relevance cannot be shown, then any other reasons that potentially bear upon a decision will be discounted, including considerations of opportunity cost. One way of thinking about the social contract test of justice is to say that someone could reasonably reject a proposed framework of priority-setting unless it contained something like the patient-relevance test in the German form.

However, even if one rejects the conclusions of the social contract argument and holds that QALY gain is always relevant, NICE social value judgements only allow for it to be only one consideration. If the NICE social value judgements were based upon an unambiguous endorsement of the QALY maximising principle, it would have a definite answer to those who question any opportunity cost argument. However, this definiteness of decision principle is only made possible by an implausible assertion, to the effect that only QALY maximisation should be decisive.

Given that NICE rejected the view that its social value judgements were purely utilitarian, it is thereby forced to the view that any social value judgement must be made up of a variety of possibly heterogeneous elements. Whether an outcome is judged better or worse than an alternative will not only depend on the QALY gain and the extent to which a technology passes a threshold test, but will also depend upon such values as fairness, legality, the reduction of health inequalities and so on. Moreover, how these values are weighed may vary from individual to individual, and there is no formula by which an overall 'super-evaluation' can be inferred from the collection of individual evaluations. Hence, it is not surprising that NICE's decisions have the object of political and policy contestation. They are caught in the Arrow problem. The paradigm builds in an underlying complexity of individual evaluations that cannot be represented in a single ordering of priorities.

Anomalies

As the NICE classical paradigm was developed and implemented, these issues of abstract principle were played out in NICE's decision-making. The result was to create decisions that were anomalous from a pure QALY maximising point of view.

One particularly striking example was in connection with the initial assessment of Lucentis, a drug aimed at the treatment of macular degeneration. Patients who lose the sight of one eye are able to adapt to their condition, so that loss of vision in one eye does not limit quality of life as much as one might be otherwise tempted to think. Hence, the initial appraisal of NICE in respect of Lucentis was that those suffering macular degeneration should be allowed to lose the sight of one eye before the treatment was administered, a view that was clearly at odds with any responsible clinical guidance for managing the condition. NICE drew back from its initial assessment citing dread risk on the part of patients as something to be avoided, but this did not stop the original initial assessment being a logically justifiable interpretation of the paradigm with which the final decision was at odds.

A second set of anomalies arose in connection with end of life considerations. In the main these arose from anti-cancer medications, like Sunitinib, Trastuzumab and Lapatinib, although they also involved Riluzole, a treatment for motor neurone disease. In each of these cases NICE was prepared to recommend a medicine, even though its cost was above the £30,000 threshold; in some cases considerably above that threshold. The justification given was that an extension of life at the end of life was especially valuable, a rationale that was clearly at odds with the principle that a QALY is a QALY is a QALY.

A third interesting anomaly was exemplified in the case of Mifamurtide, a treatment for bone cancer in the young, and used in conjunction with multi-agent chemotherapy treatments. It gave a statistically significant difference in length of survival, 7.0 years, for those treated with the medicine by comparison with a control group. Past 7.9 years, the survival period for those treated with the drug is long – around 60 years – so its benefits stretch into the future. Given the long length of survival, standard practice would have been to discount the costs and benefits by the Treasury discount rate of 3.5% per year. However, the relevant Appraisal Committee suggested that in line with the special conditions in NICE's 'Guide to the Methods of Technology Appraisal', a discount rate of 1.5% for health benefits could be used. This reduced the cost per QALY of Mifamurtide to £36,000 from an original estimate of £56,700 per year.

The common feature of these examples is that the original application of a cost-effectiveness test was revised in the light of broader considerations. In introducing these examples, I have used the term 'anomaly' deliberately. Policy analysts have taken from the philosophers of science the idea of a paradigm, defined by Kuhn (1970: 43) as 'a set of recurrent and quasi-standard illustrations of various theories in their conceptual, observational, and instrumental applications'. Kuhn used the idea to understand changes in scientific theories, including large-scale ones like the move from Ptolemaic to Copernican astronomy. But the important feature of a paradigm is that it not only provides an intellectual scheme for understanding the world, it also provides criteria relevant for defining what counts as evidence in any view of the world and what problems are taken to be significant.

For policy analysts like Hall (1993), the term paradigm was therefore valuable in understanding policy shifts like those in economic policy involving a change from post-war Keynesianism to monetarism in the 1980s. Crucially, such changes came about because of the accumulation of anomalies that have to be dealt with by policy changes. For example, demand did not shift in response to changes in interest rates in the way that Keynesian policy makers expected. This led to a first-order change in the setting of those policy instruments, for example a further resetting of interest rates. Then the instruments themselves appeared to become incapable of bringing about the ends of policy, leading to a second-order change in the choice of instruments to achieve the ends, for example the imposition of cash limits in public expenditure. Finally, a third-order change led to a reformulation of policy, as in the case of the replacement of Keynesianism by monetarism and the corresponding replacement of the goal of full employment by stable prices. As anomalies accumulate, the argument runs, so the pressure on the fundamental assumptions of the prevailing paradigm increases.

Rather than changing its paradigm wholesale, NICE's way of dealing with its anomalies was to adopt the language of 'modifiers' to considerations of pure cost-effectiveness as measured by the threshold test. The end-of-life modifier was one important example, but so too was the 'innovation' modifier, which allowed the threshold to be exceeded where a new product offered an improvement in care when improvements had not taken place in recent years (see Chapters 5 and 6). Implementing the paradigm by the application of modifiers thus remained at Hall's first-order level of change. It did not change the instruments. It certainly did not change the fundamental approach. NICE was still cleaving to the cost-effectiveness paradigm and making marginal changes, notably in the rigour of the threshold that was being applied. How far does the 2020 shift from social value judgements to principles suggest that a more fundamental paradigm change is occurring, consigning the classical paradigm to oblivion?

From values to principles?

How does the NICE (2020) statement of *Our Principles* compare with *Social Value Judgements*? From one point there does not seem to be a great difference, despite *Our Principles* opening by saying that whereas *Social Value Judgements* was developed in the context of technology appraisal, *Our Principles* is addressed to the much broader scope of work NICE had acquired over the years. Moreover, Paragraph 23 of *Our Principles* endorses the use of incremental cost-effectiveness ratio (ICER) calculations, the use of QALYs, the importance of opportunity costs as well as rejecting the rule of rescue. All these ideas are framed in the formula that the guidance and standards of NICE are addressed to 'overall population need'. Moreover, the language of 'principles' was not alien to *Social Value Judgements*, given that its subtitle was 'Principles for the Development of NICE Guidance'. Where so much is continuous, what is the significance of the change?

Clearly there has been no change from the perspective that priority-setting is a matter of achieving some overall social good rather than, for example, supporting the right to health and health care or ensuring that the high costs of individual urgent treatment are widely shared in a scheme of social solidarity. From that point of view, the ghost of the old utilitarianism lingers, being perhaps too deeply rooted in some strands of UK political culture to be changed by an administrative body (Landwehr and Klinnert, 2015). If there is change, it is not in a fundamental assumption that guided the classical paradigm. It certainly does not represent, for example, the sort of third-order change of paradigm that would take place if the UK were to adopt, say, a paradigm like Germany's in which the right to health has become important, and cost-effectiveness is replaced by the relevance of a drug to improvements in patient health (see Ettelt, 2020; Kieslich, 2012, 2020), The change is less one of substantive content than of what status NICE is claiming to possess when it makes an appraisal and how its activities fit into the policy making institutions of the state.

In claiming to express social values, the classical paradigm presented itself as taking the social point of view. As we have seen, the problems of combining a multiplicity of individual social welfare functions, each of which sought to express some social point of view, meant that any view that NICE took inevitably involved an assumption that it could speak on behalf of 'society'. *Our Principles* (note the first person plural) gives up on this idea. Instead NICE presents itself as a public agency firmly located in political and administrative processes from which it derives its authority. To look outwards, it must look upwards. Perhaps it was for this reason that it also abolished the Citizens Council, which was one partial way of addressing the Arrow problem insofar as the Citizens Council achieved unanimity.

The move from an embodiment of social values to an authoritative agency of legitimate government is not of itself an implausible view. If the ambition simply to reflect the values of society was never feasible, it makes sense for NICE to present itself as an accountable agent of government, delegated to undertake a wide but specific range of tasks, ready to consult but with the authority to make decisions in line with its mandate. The concern, however, is that this change in the way that NICE thinks of its role allows the sort of administrative discretion that undermines the ambition to provide high quality care but with a prudent use of resources. Its adoption of the principle of innovation in particular opens the door to lobbying that would privilege producer interests over patient interests and over the health needs of the population taken as a whole.

There is, perhaps, one further implication of the move from social welfare judgements to policy principles. The welfare economics on which *Social Value Judgements* rested was closely tied to a philosophical view about the logical status of value judgements, a philosophical view that was subjectivist. That view was logical positivism. According to logical positivism, value judgements were much closer to judgements of taste than to meaningful arguments. To argue about values, in the sense of providing considerations capable of determining the intellect – to use John Stuart Mill's term ([1861]1991: 135) – did not make sense on this logical positivist view, rather as one cannot really have a rational discussion about a preference for vanilla over chocolate chip nut ice cream. The widespread influence of logical positivism has waned (remaining sufferers are advised to seek counselling), but some sort of subjectivism lingers in much public discussion and some policy cultures. It may be optimistic, but one consequence of NICE's adoption of the language of principles, which must always be stated as intelligible considerations, could finally put to rest the old positivist subjectivism and replace its decision-making with reasoning according to codes of public decision-making for which there are justificatory arguments. For this particular student of the role of ideas in public policy, the wish here may be father of the thought, however.

References

Arrow, K.J. (1963) *Social Choice and Individual Values*. 2nd edn. New Haven: Yale University Press.
Barry, B. (1989) *Theories of Justice*. London: Harvester-Wheatsheaf.
Barry, B. (1995) *Justice as Impartiality*. Oxford: Oxford University Press.

Bryan, S., Williams, I., and McIver, S. (2007) 'Seeing the NICE Side of Cost-Effectiveness Analysis: A Qualitative Investigation of the Use of CEA in NICE Technology Appraisals', *Health Economics*, 16(2), pp.179–93.

Charlton, V. (2022) 'Does NICE Apply the Rule of Rescue in its Approach to Highly Specialised Technologies?', *Journal of Medical Ethics*, 48(2), pp.118–25.

Charlton, V. and Weale, A. (2021) 'Exorcising the Positivist Ghost in the Priority-Setting Machine: NICE and the Demise of the "Social Value Judgement"', *Health Economics, Policy and Law*, 16(4), pp.505–11.

Claxton, K. and Culyer, A.J. (2006) 'Wickedness or Folly? The Ethics of NICE's Decisions', *Journal of Medical Ethics*, 32(7), pp.373–77.

Coase, R. (1960) 'The Problem of Social Cost', *The Journal of Law and Economics*, 3, pp.1–44; reprinted in Coase R. (1988) *The Firm, The Market and The Law*. Chicago and London: University of Chicago Press, pp. 95–156.

Culyer, A.J. (2016) 'Cost-Effectiveness Thresholds in Health Care: A Bookshelf Guide to Their Meaning and Use', *Health Economics, Policy and Law*, 11 (4), pp.415–32.

Daniels, N. and Sabin, J. (2002) *Setting Limits Fairly: Can We Learn to Share Medical Resources?* New York: Oxford University Press.

Ettelt, S. (2020) 'Access to Treatment and the Constitutional Right to Health in Germany: A Triumph of Hope over Evidence?', *Health Economics, Policy and Law*, 15(1), pp.30–42.

Gauthier, D. (1979) 'David Hume, Contractarian', *Philosophical Review*, 88(1), pp.3–38.

Hall, P.A. (1993) 'Policy Paradigms, Social Learning and the State', *Comparative Politics*, 25(3), pp.275–96.

Harsanyi, J.C. (1955) 'Individualistic Ethics, and Interpersonal Comparisons of Utility', *Journal of Political Economy*, 63(4), pp.309–21.

Kieslich, K. (2012) 'Social Values and Health Priority Setting in Germany', *Journal of Health Organization and Management*, 26(3), pp.374–83.

Kieslich, K. (2020) 'Paradigms in Operation: Explaining Pharmaceutical Benefit Assessments in England and Germany', *Health Economics, Policy and Law*, 15(3), pp.370–85.

Kuhn, T.S. (1970) *The Structure of Scientific Revolutions*. 2nd edn. Chicago: University of Chicago Press.

Landwehr, C. and Klinnert, D. (2015) 'Value Congruence in Healthcare Priority Setting: Social Values, Institutions and Decisions', *Health Economics, Policy and Law*, 10(2), pp.113–32.

Menzel, P. (2007) 'Allocation of Scarce Resources' in Rhodes, R., Francis, L.P., and Silvers, A. (eds), *The Blackwell Guide to Medical Ethics*. Oxford: Blackwell, pp.305–22.

Mill, J.S. (1861) 'Utilitarianism', in *On Liberty and Other Essays*, edited with an Introduction by Gray, J. (1991) Oxford: Oxford University Press, pp.129–201.

NICE (2008) *Social Value Judgements*. 2nd edn. London: NICE.

NICE (2020) *Our Principles: The Principles that Guide the Development of NICE Guidance and Standards*. London: NICE.

Rawlins, M. and Culyer, A.J. (2004) 'National Institute for Clinical Excellence and its Value Judgements', *British Medical Journal*, 329, pp.224–27.

Rawls, J. (1999) *A Theory of Justice*. Revised edn. Cambridge, MA: Harvard University Press.

Rid, A. (2009) 'Justice and Procedure: How Does "Accountability for Reasonableness" Result in Fair Limit-Setting Decisions?', *Journal of Medical Ethics*, 35(1), pp.12–16.

Rumbold, B., Weale, A., Rid, A., Wilson, J., and Littlejohns, P. (2017) 'Public Reasoning and Health Care Priority Setting: The Case of NICE', *Kennedy Institute of Ethics Journal*, 27(1), pp.107–34.

Scanlon, T.M. (1982) 'Contractualism and Utilitarianism' in Sen, A. and Williams, B. (eds), *Utilitarianism and Beyond*. Cambridge: Cambridge University Press, pp.101–28.

Scanlon, T.M. (1998) *What We Owe to Each Other*. Cambridge, MA and London: Belknap Press.

Sen, A. (1970) *Collective Choice and Social Welfare*. San Francisco: Holden-Day.

Weale, A. (2018) *The Will of the People: A Modern Myth*. Cambridge: Polity Press.

Weale, A. (2020) *Modern Social Contract Theory*. Oxford: Oxford University Press.

Williams, A. (1985) 'Economics of Coronary Bypass Grafting', *British Medical Journal*, 291, pp.326–29.

Williams, A. (2004) *What Could Be Nicer than NICE?* London: Office of Health Economics. Available at: https://www.ohe.org/publications/what-could-be-nicer-nice/ (Accessed 4 June 2023).

5   Innovation, values and NICE's changing societal role

Victoria Charlton

Origins: the need for a legitimate gatekeeper

NICE was created at a time when Britney Spears was top of the UK charts, the Euro currency was in its first weeks of circulation and a recently impeached Bill Clinton was US President. Apple's release of its first iPhone was still eight years away and the human genome project was yet to fully sequence an entire human chromosome (NHGRI, 2022). NICE was a product of its time and that time was a very different one to now.

It is generally accepted that three concerns about the state of the NHS in the mid-1990s were influential in laying the foundations for NICE's establishment (Syrett, 2003; Crinson, 2004; Timmins, Rawlins and Appleby, 2016; Atkinson and Sheard, 2020). The first arose from intense public debate about the 'postcode lottery': a phenomenon in which delegation of decision-making to local budget holders led to geographical differences in access to NHS treatments. The second related to anxiety about the quality of NHS care following a series of high-profile scandals, including the arrest of Dr Harold Shipman, the discovery of excess cardiac deaths at the Bristol Royal Infirmary and the inappropriate treatment of human tissues at Alder Hey Hospital. The third was recognition of the growing financial pressure faced by the NHS following several years of modest spending increases under the Conservative government, combined with the emergence of an increasing array of new and expensive health technologies and the expectation of a growing, ageing and ever more demanding patient population (Wanless, 2002; King's Fund, 2005; Rodwin, 2021).

These concerns meant that, in the run up to the 1997 General Election, the NHS was a key topic of national debate. While financial pressures and concerns about quality highlighted the need for the NHS to utilise its resources efficiently, the highly visible – and, to many, patently unjust – practice of postcode prescribing highlighted the equally important need to distribute NHS resources in a way that could be defended as fair.

The question of how NHS resources should be 'rationed' when demand outstrips supply was (and remains), however, an unappealing one for politicians to

DOI: 10.4324/9781003501268-5

engage with; a fact that had recently been underlined by the case of beta interferon. Licenced in 1995, beta interferon was a promising but expensive new treatment for multiple sclerosis (MS) – a serious condition thought to affect around 70,000 patients in England (Crinson, 2004; Timmins, Rawlins and Appleby, 2016). Clinical trials suggested that the drug reduced the frequency and severity of attacks in patients with the relapsing-remitting form of MS, but evidence for its long-term effectiveness was uncertain and its potential impact on NHS budgets was huge (Crinson, 2004). The Government, working with the NHS Executive, therefore advised heath authorities to manage the financial impact of beta interferon by limiting its use. But while eligible patients in some areas were granted access to the drug, similar patients in other areas were not, resulting in some local decisions coming under legal challenge. Public discontent at the Government's handling of the situation was significant (Crinson, 2004).

As this drama played out, a Labour party led by Tony Blair was elected on the back of a promise to 'save the NHS' (Labour Party, 1997). The new Government pledged to improve quality while also addressing concerns about fairness, promising that access to interventions would be based 'on need and need alone' (ibid.). Another key theme of Blair's 'New Labour' was a commitment to rational decision-making and policies 'shaped by evidence' (Cabinet Office, 1999). 'What counts is what works', it declared (ibid.), and recent advances in health evaluation and technology assessment carried the promise of an evidence-based approach to establishing 'what works' in efficiently distributing healthcare resources.

The creation of NICE in April 1999 thus addressed both a practical and a political problem. As a source of centralised guidance on the NHS's use of new and existing health technologies, NICE would give practical advice to the health service, promoting the effective use of limited resources while ensuring 'greater local consistency' in access to interventions (Department of Health, 1997). As an independent body whose decisions were demonstrably evidence-based, it was also positioned as a morally legitimate 'gatekeeper' to the NHS, 'scientifically depoliticising the rationing debate' (Syrett, 2003) and protecting the Government from the political risk associated with making unpopular – but necessary – priority-setting decisions.

Securing a claim to legitimacy

NICE's political architects intended the Institute to act as an 'independent, hard-nosed, authoritative, evidence-based' decision-maker (Milburn, 2000, in Syrett, 2003), setting healthcare priorities on society's behalf. NICE's formal remit was thus to provide 'clear, authoritative guidance on clinical and cost-effectiveness' so that interventions which offered good value to the NHS could be 'actively promoted', while 'protect[ing] patients from new interventions' for which the available evidence was 'inadequate' (Department of Health, 1998).

NICE's formal establishment gave it legal and political authority to fulfil this role. But to be effective it also had to secure a moral mandate to act on society's behalf, thereby protecting itself from the fallout that would inevitably arise from unpopular decisions. NICE's early rejection of the flu drug zanamivir (Relenza) in 1999 demonstrated its committees' willingness to make such decisions. But this case also highlighted NICE's vulnerability to political and commercial pressure and the critical public and media attention that its decisions – particularly those that were negative – could expect to receive. From 2002, therefore, NICE took more active steps to establish and demonstrate its status as a morally legitimate decision-maker.[1]

Reasonableness and fairness: the pillars of NICE's normative approach

These steps centred on publicly articulating a consistent approach to decision-making that could be shown to be both reasonable and fair.[2]

NICE's commitment to reasonableness drew heavily on its 'evidence-based' identity and was grounded on the principle that NICE should show 'methodological robustness' (later, 'scientific rigour') in using evidence as the basis for its decision-making (NICE, 2005; NICE, 2008). This provided a sound footing from which to defend its decisions as rational, and allowed NICE to maintain an aspect of scientific impartiality that could be useful in justifying unpopular outcomes.

Given the historical context from which NICE arose, however, it was not enough for its decisions to be reasonable; it was also essential that they be accepted as fair. NICE sought to show that its decisions met this requirement through reference to two complementary frameworks.

The first, 'accountability for reasonableness' (AfR), was a procedural framework developed by American academics Norman Daniels and James Sabin in response to the comparable 'legitimacy problem' faced by US health insurers seeking to place limits on their coverage of medical interventions (Daniels and Sabin, 1997). It set out four conditions that were considered necessary and sufficient for procedural justice to be served: (1) both the decisions made and the grounds for reaching them must be made public ('publicity'); (2) those grounds

---

1 A distinction is drawn here between justice and moral legitimacy. While justice is taken to relate to something's moral quality, legitimacy is taken to relate to the moral authority of the state to compel people to accept its laws and judgements. Thus, a decision made by NICE could be defended as just but might not possess the quality of moral legitimacy if, for example, it is beyond NICE's remit to make such a decision. It is also acknowledged that legitimacy draws on other sources of normativity as well as morality; for example, political legitimacy, legal legitimacy, constitutional legitimacy and so on. See (Hickey, 2022).

2 A third value underpinning NICE decision-making is a commitment to lawfulness; however, this aspect of NICE's approach is discussed in detail in Chapter 9 and so will not be considered here.

must be ones that fair-minded people would agree are relevant in the particular context ('relevance'); (3) there must be opportunities for challenging and revising decisions and resolving disputes ('appeal and revision'), and (4) there must be measures in place to ensure compliance with the first three conditions ('enforcement'). As long as a priority-setter could demonstrate that its procedures met these conditions – as NICE broadly claimed to do (NICE, 2005) – then proponents of AfR argued that both its approach and its decisions should be accepted as fair.

In the last two decades, AfR has been widely adopted amongst healthcare priority-setters and has demonstrated its usefulness as a standard for procedural fairness (Daniels and Sabin, 2008). But commentators have challenged the claim that AfR's conditions are sufficient to ensure that decisions are just (Friedman, 2008; Lauridsen and Lippert-Rasmussen, 2009; Rid, 2009; Ford, 2015; Rand, 2016). From a practical perspective, AfR's relatively vague requirement that decisions be based on 'relevant' reasons also left space for outcomes that might be perceived as inconsistent. In attempting to demonstrate the fairness of its approach, NICE therefore set out a second framework that specified the substantive grounds on which decisions would generally be made.

Central to these is consideration of a technology's cost-effectiveness: that is, 'the value of the treatment relative to alternative uses of resources in the NHS' (HC Debate, 2 December 1999). Under this 'opportunity-cost' based approach,[3] NICE indicated that it would generally only recommend a new technology if evidence demonstrated that it was cost-effective compared to alternative uses: a judgement explicitly defined, from 2004 onwards, according to a threshold of £20,000 to £30,000 per quality-adjusted life-year (QALY).[4] However, NICE recognised that efficiency is not the NHS's only normative concern and therefore allowed its committees to consider other relevant reasons in deciding whether a particular technology should be made available. Thus, a committee might recommend a relatively cost-ineffective or unproven technology if it believed that other factors – such as the severity of the condition being treated, or the magnitude of the benefit potentially offered – were sufficiently strong to justify the associated opportunity cost.

This substantive understanding of fairness closely reflected the gatekeeper role assigned to NICE at the time of its establishment and its undertaking to 'promote the appropriate use of those interventions which offer good value to patients

---

3 Opportunity cost is defined as the benefits foregone when one alternative is chosen over another.
4 The QALY is a universal quantitative measure of a technology's effect on both quantity and quality of life. The former is measured in life-years and the latter on a 0–1 scale, with the two figures being multiplied to produce an estimated QALY gain (or loss). The cost/QALY is therefore a measure of the amount of health delivered per pound spent by the NHS, compared with current treatment. Generally, if this exceeds £20,000–£30,000/QALY, a technology will not be considered to be cost-effective.

and to discourage the use of those which do not' (NICE, 1999). It also aligned closely with NICE's commitment to evidence-based medicine and its broadly technocratic conception of what constitutes a reasonable decision. Perhaps most importantly, this approach could be defended as ethically sound (Rumbold et al., 2017) and was informed by the deliberations of NICE's Citizens Council, a representative body that provided societal insight on normative issues relevant to NICE's work (Rawlins, 2005; Davies, Barnett and Wetherell, 2006).

As such, from the mid-2000s, NICE openly committed itself to following this approach and proactively communicated it to both clinical and lay audiences (Rawlins and Culyer, 2004; Rawlins, 2005; NICE, 2005; Pearson and Rawlins, 2005). In doing so, it provided itself with a firm basis for justifying its decisions and for asserting its authority as a morally legitimate priority-setter.

The evolution of NICE's normative approach

Of course, this approach was not without its critics: some disagreed with procedural aspects while others considered it to be substantively flawed (Smith, 2000; Cookson, McDaid and Maynard, 2001; Maynard, Bloor and Freemantle, 2004; Harris, 2005a; Harris, 2005b; Harris, 2006; Harris, 2007; Quigley, 2007; Schlander, 2008). But it was logically and morally coherent and could – when needed – be robustly defended by those at NICE's helm (Rawlins and Dillon, 2005; Claxton and Culyer, 2006; Claxton and Culyer, 2007; Claxton and Culyer, 2008; Stevens et al., 2012). It was also, at the time, closely aligned with government priorities and Labour's promise to control NHS costs while improving quality and tackling perceived sources of inequity (Department of Health, 1998).

However, the controversial nature of NICE's role and the changing environment in which it has operated over the last 25 years have subjected it to substantial social, political, commercial and operational pressures. Over time, these pressures have driven NICE to evolve, creating a clear distinction between the approach articulated in the early 2000s and that employed by the Institute today. In the language of Chapter 6, NICE has engaged in both means-improvement and what its proponents would likely describe as values-improvement.

This 'values-improvement' has been driven by three key trends.[5] The first relates to NICE's changing conception of fairness and the extent to which concern for opportunity cost has become secondary to other considerations. The second relates to the idea of reasonableness and the reduced evidential burden

---

5 The first two of these three trends emerge from the findings of Charlton (2020). The third has been observed through more recent empirical work (Charlton and DiStefano, 2024).

now placed on the technologies recommended by NICE. And the third relates to NICE's willingness to revise its judgements in response to commercial negotiation. Together, these trends, driven by a shift in values, contribute to a major shift in NICE's societal role: from that of NHS gatekeeper to that of facilitator in securing the NHS access to new technologies.

Benefitting the few at the cost to the many

Since its establishment, NICE's conception of fairness has given regard to the interests of both those known patients whose health will be improved through access to a new technology, and those unknown patients whose health will suffer due to the allocation of resources away from alternative uses. In balancing the interests of these groups, it has long considered a threshold of £20,000 to £30,000 to be the 'most appropriate' reflection of NHS opportunity cost and therefore an indication that a technology is likely to be cost-effective (NICE, 2013).[6]

This threshold was never intended to function as an absolute rule: NICE has always acknowledged that technologies costing less than £20,000/QALY may sometimes be rejected and those costing more than £30,000/QALY recommended, if justified by the circumstances (NICE, 2004). Indeed, a wide range of factors aside from cost-effectiveness have been shown to influence NICE decision-making (Charlton, 2022b). But in the early years of NICE's work such deviations were relatively rare and were generally based on committees' consideration of the exceptional features of particular cases (Shah et al., 2013).

This case-based approach began to change in the late 2000s. At the time, NICE's gatekeeping role was facing challenge from the increasing number of costly technologies – particularly cancer drugs – receiving regulatory approval from the European Medicines Agency (Timmins, Rawlins and Appleby, 2016), many of which did not meet NICE's £20,000 to £30,000/QALY threshold. Following NICE's failure to promptly recommend several cancer drugs in the mid-2000s, a national debate was sparked concerning whether NHS patients with the means to pay 'out-of-pocket' for treatments not approved by NICE should be allowed to do so. The incumbent Labour government was ideologically opposed to such 'top-up' arrangements but, in the face of strong opposition from patients and families – and under threat of judicial review – it commissioned an independent expert to consider the issue (Chalkidou, 2012; Timmins, Rawlins and Appleby, 2016). The resulting 2008 report, *Improving Access to Medicines for NHS Patients*, concluded that top-ups should generally be prohibited, but

---

6 NICE continues to use this figure as its standard cost-effectiveness threshold, but recent evidence suggests that this considerably underestimates the amount of health displaced from the NHS to fund new technologies. See Chapter 2 and Martin et al. (2021).

advised that NICE should show more willingness to recommend high-cost treatments for late-stage cancer (Richards, 2008).

NICE's response was to formally alter its approach such that QALYs derived from technologies that extended the life of terminally ill patients would routinely be valued more highly than QALYs experienced by other patients, in effect increasing the cost-effectiveness threshold for this group (NICE, 2009). The political motivation for this change was clear but the so-called 'end-of-life' rules appeared ethically problematic (Cookson, 2013; Fleck, 2018) and their real-world effect was to reduce the amount of health that could be delivered from the NHS's limited budget (Collins and Latimer, 2013).[7] Subsequent changes that prioritised the needs of other groups were similarly questioned (O'Mahony and Paulden, 2014; Paulden et al., 2014; Charlton, 2022a) and, in some cases, appeared to conflict with the views of NICE's Citizens Council (NICE Citizens Council, 2004; NICE Citizens Council, 2008a; NICE Citizens Council, 2008b; NICE Citizens Council, 2009). Such modifications potentially undermined NICE's perceived moral legitimacy, but they also signalled a fundamental shift in NICE's conception of fairness. While NICE had historically adopted a utilitarian view that sought to avoid the use of inefficient technologies in order to improve health at a population level, its new approach was implicitly prioritarian, and accepted that a substantial opportunity cost may need to be tolerated by the many if the highly valued benefits of certain new technologies were to be realised by the few.

Giving new technologies the benefit of the doubt

At the time of its establishment, as well as improving efficiency, NICE was intended to improve the quality of NHS care by accelerating access to treatments 'known to work' and by ensuring that patients could be 'assured of the benefit' likely to be derived from new technologies (Department of Health, 1998). This placed the burden of evidence firmly on those technologies undergoing appraisal, which were required to actively justify their adoption by clearly demonstrating their clinical and cost-effectiveness compared with existing interventions.

As a consequence of this requirement, in its early years NICE took a conservative approach to managing the uncertainty that inevitably surrounds new technologies, expressing a 'strong preference' for evidence derived from randomised controlled trials and advising that its committees 'should not recommend an intervention if there is no evidence, or not enough evidence, on which to make a clear decision' (NICE, 2004: 11; NICE, 2008: 16). In subsequent years, however, global regulatory and commercial standards have reduced reliance on large

---

7 It is estimated that, between 2009 and 2011, technologies recommended under the end-of-life rules delivered 12,401 QALYs per year to late-stage NHS cancer patients. The opportunity cost to other NHS users was estimated at between 18,330 and 27,496 QALYs, generating a net loss to the NHS of between 5,929 and 15,095 QALYs. See (Collins and Latimer, 2013).

clinical trials, in favour of policies intended to accelerate patient access to innovative treatments (Davis and Abraham, 2013). NICE is therefore now regularly faced with the problem of how to respond when a promising new technology, approved by the regulator, lacks the evidence necessary to support a confident conclusion about its clinical- and cost-effectiveness.

As part of its commitment to acting reasonably, NICE would historically have been expected to simply reject such technologies in order to protect patients and the health system from the risks associated with adopting unproven and possibly poor value treatments. However, this response – which formed part of NICE's *raison d'être* in 1999 – has increasingly been perceived as unacceptable to both patients and politicians.[8] This has left NICE reluctant to reject promising technologies on the grounds of uncertainty alone. In attempting to maintain coherence between its approach and its decisions, NICE has thus altered its conception of reasonableness to reduce the burden of evidence under which new technologies are placed. This has been achieved through a variety of mechanisms, all of which have allowed NICE to maintain its commitment to 'evidence-based' decision-making. Periodic updates to NICE's technical guides have included new material on the use of non-randomised, non-controlled studies and on statistical modelling techniques that can help to bridge gaps in the available evidence, in what NICE presents as its new 'comprehensive approach to assessing the best evidence that is available' (Charlton, 2020; NICE, 2020d). More recently, NICE has specified certain types of technology that might reasonably warrant recommendation despite displaying 'a higher degree of uncertainty' than would usually be considered acceptable – for example, 'innovative and complex' technologies and drugs for rare diseases (NICE, 2022d: 172). The most prominent development along this trajectory, however, has been the expansion of NICE's use of managed access arrangements: commercial deals in which the NHS agrees to provisionally adopt a technology while evidence collection continues.

Used occasionally since the mid-2000s, managed access arrangements became the standard mode of adoption for drugs recommended via the Cancer Drugs Fund (CDF) in 2016[9] and are now a regular feature of NICE appraisal. Aimed at facilitating NHS access to uncertain technologies, they are positioned by NICE as a reasonable response to cases in which a technology has 'the plausible potential to be cost-effective' but for which existing evidence is relatively weak (NICE, 2022d: 177). During the period of managed access the technology is funded by the NHS at a discounted price, before being reappraised by NICE

---

8 As evidenced, for example, by public and political debate surrounding NICE's appraisal of lumacaftor–ivacaftor (Orkambi) for cystic fibrosis and nusinersen (Spinraza) for spinal muscular atrophy.

9 The CDF is a source of ring-fenced public funding for cancer drugs unable to secure a full recommendation from NICE. It was established in 2011 and has been administered in part by NICE since 2016.

following further evidence collection. At the time of writing, 33 treatments were available through managed access, with an annual budget of £680 million set aside to fund these types of arrangements (NICE, 2023a).

Through such developments NICE's conception of reasonableness has evolved away from one centred on scientific rigour and a technology's need to demonstrate clinical- and cost-effectiveness, to one that is far more tolerant of uncertainty and risk. Historically willing to reject technologies that failed to meet its high evidential requirements, NICE is increasingly happy to offer some new technologies the benefit of the doubt – at least until evidence of cost-*ineffectiveness* emerges.

From 'Yes' or 'No', to 'Is that your best offer?'

The cost-effectiveness of a new technology depends not just on its clinical-effectiveness, but also on its price, with even fairly ineffective technologies potentially meeting NICE's £20,000 to £30,000/QALY threshold if the costs are sufficiently low. But price negotiation does not form part of NICE's legal remit and was something that, at the time of its establishment, Health Minister Frank Dobson felt should remain 'separate' from NICE technology appraisal, to prevent decisions from being 'sull[ied]' through exposure to commercial discussions' (Timmins, Rawlins and Appleby, 2016: 69).[10] As such, the original NICE appraisal process did not include any formal occasion for manufacturers to revise their price – and thereby improve their technology's cost-effectiveness – following initial submission.

The advent of managed access and other confidential pricing arrangements, however, have introduced several formal opportunities for negotiation, allowing manufacturers to revise their commercial offer as necessary to secure a recommendation. One such opportunity follows a committee's provisional decision to reject a technology, having expressed its views about its value and indicated what it believes to be the technology's likely cost/QALY. A common pattern is therefore for a company to revise its offer to the NHS (or, on occasion, the evidence submitted to NICE) in light of these views, with the intention of bringing the cost/QALY within – just – the range likely to be considered acceptable by the committee. In this scenario, while NICE plays an important role in providing the NHS with leverage for commercial discussions, the final decision is, to some extent, in the manufacturer's hands; every technology has its price, and it is up to the manufacturer to decide whether it is willing to offer the price that the committee likely requires for the threshold to be met. A side-effect of this pattern is that the final cost/QALY

---

10 This remained NICE's position for many years and the Institute was expressly prohibited from negotiating until 2019 under the terms of the 2014 Pharmaceutical Price Regulation Scheme. See (Department of Health and ABPI, 2013).

on which NICE's recommendation is based is often publicly redacted because of the confidential nature of the agreed upon price discount (Bullement et al., 2019).

This willingness to turn a 'no' into a 'yes' further to negotiation offers a sensible strategy if NICE's goal is to recommend as many technologies as possible at a price that is acceptable to the NHS. However, it is not the approach of an 'independent, hard-nosed, authoritative, evidence-based' gatekeeper (Milburn, 2000, in Syrett, 2003) whose role is to 'protect' the health service from interventions for which there is 'inadequate evidence' (Department of Health, 1998). The central position that NICE now takes in the negotiation process is therefore indicative of its new role, not as gatekeeper, but as facilitator, responsible for working with industry and the health system to bring about the adoption of new technologies.

Together, these three trends – illustrated through the case in Box 5.1 – have thus contributed to a major shift in NICE's societal role: a shift that has substantial implications for the way that NHS resources are distributed. But on what grounds might this change in NICE's fundamental goals and approach be justified?

The answer appears to lie in the concept of innovation.

Box 5.1   Illustrating the three trends: the case of atezolizumab

Atezolizumab (Tecentriq) is a cancer immunotherapy assessed by NICE in 2019–2020, whose appraisal illustrates the Institute's willingness to recommend 'innovative' technologies beyond the usual cost-effectiveness threshold, based on uncertain evidence and further to commercial negotiation. It is presented as an example of the type of recommendation made possible by the evolution of NICE's approach over recent years.

Atezolizumab is a monoclonal antibody designed to attach to a protein called PD-L1, an immune 'checkpoint' that modulates activity by a part of the immune system that would otherwise attack cancer cells. By binding to PD-L1, atezolizumab is thought to reduce its effects and thereby enhance the body's immune response to certain cancers (European Medicines Agency, 2023).

Atezolizumab gained regulatory approval as a treatment for triple-negative breast cancer in August 2019 (European Medicines Agency, 2019). This approval was based on the findings of the IMpassion130 trial, a double-blind randomised controlled trial that compared atezolizumab plus nab-paclitaxel (a taxane-based chemotherapy) against placebo plus nab-paclitaxel in 902 breast cancer patients (Schmid et al., 2018). The trial showed that patients who received atezolizumab lived for an average of 7.2 months without their disease progressing, compared with 5.5 months in the control group: a statistically significant improvement in progression free survival. However, the difference in overall survival between these two groups – that is, the length of time that patients actually lived following initiation of treatment – was not statistically significant (ibid.). According to the trial protocol, this finding should have precluded any further analysis of how effective atezolizumab was in particular subgroups of patients, because the trial was not powered to test this hypothesis (clinicaltrials.gov., 2017). However, a subgroup analysis was nevertheless conducted and appeared to show that PD-L1-positive patients who received the drug survived for 25 months compared with 15.5 months in the control group (Schmid et al., 2018).

In its assessment of atezolizumab, the NICE appraisal committee noted that there were several 'areas of uncertainty' regarding the drug's clinical- and cost-effectiveness. The treatment used as the control arm for the IMpassion130 study 'is not routinely used in UK clinical practice' and the company's attempt to indirectly compare atezolizumab with current NHS care was 'not reliable and lacks face validity' (NICE, 2020a). The committee also recognised that the trial protocol did not allow for subgroup analysis. However, it accepted the conjectural results of the company's 'informal' analysis and concluded that atezolizumab 'could increase overall survival' (ibid.). As a result, it judged that the drug met NICE's criteria for consideration as an end-of-life technology and applied a cost-effectiveness threshold of £50,000/QALY.

Despite this enhanced threshold, NICE initially rejected atezolizumab in October 2019 on the grounds that it was not cost-effective (NICE, 2019). However, 'following consultation, the company updated its commercial arrangement' and atezolizumab was subsequently recommended in July 2020 (NICE, 2020a). In the press release announcing this decision, NICE described atezolizumab as a 'breakthrough treatment' which evidence suggests 'can increase overall survival by around 9.5 months' (NICE, 2020c).

Since then, results have been published for IMpassion131, a follow-up study that was underway at the time of NICE's appraisal (Miles et al., 2021). Also a double-blind randomised controlled trial, IMpassion131 tested atezolizumab plus paclitaxel (another taxane-based chemotherapy) against placebo plus paclitaxel in 651 patients, and was specifically designed to test the hypothesis that atezolizumab would be more effective in the PD-L1 subgroup. It found, however, that treatment with atezolizumab did not improve progression free survival or overall survival in either the PD-L1 subgroup or the wider trial population. Indeed, evidence suggests that atezolizumab may actually reduce overall survival in both groups (Miles et al., 2021). The reasons for this finding are unclear and remain the subject of debate (Van Wambeke and Gyawali, 2021).

At the time of writing, atezolizumab continues to be available through the NHS. It is estimated that around 600 breast cancer patients will be eligible for treatment each year, at an undiscounted list price of £39,981 per treatment course (NICE, 2020c). The total cost of the drug to the NHS, and the estimated cost/QALY used for NICE decision-making, remain confidential.

NICE and innovation

Innovation is a notoriously difficult concept to pin down (Kennedy, 2009) and, despite its regular reference to the importance of innovation, NICE itself has shied away from offering any clear definition. NICE's online glossary, for example, which contains around 400 entries for terms relevant to NICE's work, does not include an entry for innovation (NICE, 2020b) and the term is also not defined in any of NICE's technical guides, its strategy, its charter or its statement of principles.

Nevertheless, supporting the NHS's uptake of innovation has always constituted part of NICE's formal function, albeit historically as an ancillary goal, secondary to that of ensuring that the technologies adopted by the NHS are clinically- and cost-effective. At the time of NICE's establishment, this commitment was limited to acting in a way that was 'sympathetic' to the benefits of 'encouraging innovation of good value to patients' (NICE, n.d.), as acknowledged in NICE's social value judgements (NICE, 2008; NICE, 2005). Supporting innovation did not, however, then comprise one of NICE's key principles and it appeared to carry relatively little weight in decision-making in the early to mid-2000s (Charlton and Rid, 2019). As one contemporary editorial observed, in its early years NICE was often willing to put 'the 'no' in innovation' by rejecting novel drugs if they failed to meet its criteria for approval (Nat. Biotechnol., 2009).

This has since changed, with support for innovation now occupying a prominent position in NICE's identity and approach. Since 2012, consideration of a technology's 'innovativeness' has been shown to play a meaningful role in the majority of NICE appraisals and has been regularly used to justify recommending a technology above the usual cost-effectiveness threshold (Charlton and Rid, 2019). In 2020, 'support[ing] innovation' was included for the first time in NICE's statement of key principles (NICE, 2020d) and innovation is also central to NICE's 2021–2026 strategic plan, which is framed not around matters of cost-effectiveness, but around the need 'to embrace innovation by speeding up access to new and effective treatments, practices and technologies' (NICE, 2021a). Recent changes to NICE's methods are similarly framed as adaptations designed to 'give patients earlier access to innovative new treatments', by allowing committees 'greater flexibility' in their judgements about cost-effectiveness and by considering a 'broader evidence base' in attempting to understand a technology's likely effects (NICE, 2022e). Thus, NICE has celebrated its recommendation of all 15 recently appraised breast cancer drugs, for example, as evidence of its work 'driving innovation into the hands of clinicians' (NICE, 2022g), despite the apparently marginal effectiveness of some of these drugs (see Box 5.1). Press releases announcing these and other decisions frequently likewise celebrate the 'innovative' (NICE, 2022a; NICE, 2022c; NICE, 2022h; NICE, 2022i), 'ground-breaking' (NICE, 2023b), 'cutting-edge' (NICE, 2022f), 'game-changing' (NICE, 2022g), 'pioneering' (NICE, 2023b) or 'breakthrough' (NICE, 2020c) nature of such technologies.

Many new medicines do, of course, offer significant benefits to patients and some do so in a way that is genuinely original and highly cost-effective. However, the patented status of the technologies appraised by NICE means that all have some claim to novelty and NICE's support for innovation has become increasingly decoupled from a technology's ability to demonstrate its value over existing alternatives. Formal articulations of NICE's role now refer, without caveat, to the 'desirability of promoting innovation' (Health and Social Care Act 2012, s.233(1)(c)), despite many 'innovative' technologies not meeting NICE's usual standard of cost-effectiveness. This is reflected in the recent establishment of the Innovative Medicines Fund: a managed access fund intended to replicate the CDF model by providing provisional NHS access to technologies that cannot reliably demonstrate their cost-effectiveness based on the available evidence (NICE/NHS England, 2022).

But why is NICE so concerned about supporting innovation?

As detailed in Chapter 6, the ethical rationales for assigning specific value to innovation within NICE's existing approach appear weak. If NICE's primary role is to promote population health, then what seems relevant to decision-making is the health benefits that a technology generates, not the novelty of its pharmacological mechanism or the significance of the science that underpins it. If a technology offers a large health gain compared with existing treatment then, under NICE's original approach, it should be – and would be – recognised as valuable, however innovative it may be. Similar arguments can be applied to other types of benefit. If a technology offers health gains that are not well captured by the cost/QALY metric, or if it offers other types of benefit valued by society, then this should be taken into consideration, irrespective of the technology's innovativeness. An alternative approach would be to argue that the good associated with innovation is inherent rather than instrumental; that is, that innovation is valuable in itself, whatever its effects, perhaps as a proxy for 'human progress' or some other fundamental good. But NICE has made no attempt to present this argument and such a position would not align well with the goals of the NHS, which are primarily focused on promoting population health rather than furthering scientific knowledge or progress in the life sciences. Other more ethically robust rationales may of course exist, but these have not been put forward by NICE, which has tended to justify its support for innovation with reference to the health benefits that innovative technologies can purportedly generate (NICE, 2021a).

It is therefore to other, non-ethics-based explanations that we must speculatively turn in seeking to understand why NICE's approach has evolved to centre on the promotion of innovation.

Industrial strategy, the technological imperative and path dependency

Like NICE itself, the concept of innovation has evolved over time. Associated historically with subversive notions of disruptive change and revolution, it has since taken on new meanings and today carries strongly positive connotations of progress and utility (Godin, 2016). In UK public policy, as in other spheres, innovation has come to be framed, since the late 1990s, as an instrumental asset; as an 'essential' resource if the economic and social challenges of the 21st century are to be met (Osborne and Brown, 2011).

In this context, NICE's early sympathy for innovation is understandable, particularly given the medical benefits expected to arise from contemporary scientific advances such as the cultivation of embryonic stem cells and the sequencing of the human genome. But the political desire to foster innovation has intensified in the last two decades and, in the UK, innovation is now presented not just as the remedy for a variety of social and economic ills, but as a key driver of economic growth. This is reflected in recent industrial policy and, in particular, in successive government efforts to support and expand the UK life sciences sector.

Focus on the life sciences as a vital component of the 'knowledge economy' and as a key driver of economic growth has gained momentum over NICE's lifetime, with a host of developments in the early 2010s firmly establishing the sector's political importance. The Government's dedicated Office for Life Sciences (OLS), created in 2009, was tasked with 'safeguarding the future of our life sciences industry', in part by considering 'how the NHS can be more effective as a champion of innovation' and by developing 'possible ways of getting medicines onto the market faster' (PMLive, 2009). Plans for an 'innovation pass' that would allow selected products to bypass NICE appraisal were announced shortly afterwards (Department of Health, 2009; Nat. Biotechnol., 2009) and were followed in 2011 by a 'Strategy for UK Life Sciences' that outlined a detailed agenda for reforms aimed at 'overcoming barriers and creating incentives for the promotion of healthcare innovation' (Department for Business,

Innovation and Skills, 2011). Five years later, the Government's commissioned *Accelerated Access Review* made a suite of further recommendations intended 'to speed up access to innovative drugs' (Taylor and Bell, 2016). Further major life science policies followed in 2017 (Bell, 2017) and 2018 (Office for Life Sciences, 2018) and have since been joined by a new *Life Sciences Vision,* which recognises the sector as 'among the most valuable and strategically important in the UK economy' (HM Government, 2021). The NHS – no longer just a driver of population health – is presented by this Vision as potentially 'the country's most powerful driver of innovation' (ibid.: 4).

In light of this deluge of policy, it is not surprising that NICE has ceased trying to put the 'no' in innovation. Despite its independent status, the recent political environment has made it extremely difficult for NICE to reject promising technologies without bringing itself into direct conflict with government policy and what has been a major economic priority for successive regimes. It has therefore chosen instead to acknowledge its own potential 'to make a contribution to supporting a thriving life sciences sector' (NICE, 2017: 1) and, it seems, has modified its approach accordingly.

This appetite for new technology is not just politically and economically driven: society itself seems vulnerable to a deep sociological, perhaps psychological drive to embrace innovation. The technological imperative – the sense that if scientific developments mean that we *can* do something, it follows that we *should* do it (Park, 2007) – has long been an element of society's relationship with innovation and, in healthcare in particular, 'technology has become the paradigm of effective action' (Hofmann, 2002: 677; Tymstra, 1989). As early as the 1980s, it was recognised that medical technologies, which 'began as simple tools and purely effective extensions of the physician's personal approach to the patient' have since become 'intrinsic, self-propagating, requisite and almost autonomous elements of today's biomedicine' (Wolf and Berle, 1981: 125). Society as a whole, and the medical establishment in particular, like NICE, finds it hard to put the 'no' in innovation.

When faced with a new technology, experience shows that we want to believe that it works and are sometimes willing to suspend disbelief if doing so allows us to address an otherwise intractable problem (Hong, 2022). The high price of such technologies – and the opportunity cost associated with their use – does not appear to dampen our enthusiasm and may actually enhance our perception of their effectiveness. In a small but intriguing study published in 2015, 12 patients with Parkinson's disease were randomised to receive either an 'expensive' or 'cheap' new treatment, both of which were actually saline injections. Blinded assessments of motor function and MRI scans of brain activity later showed that while both placebo treatments improved symptoms, greater benefit was seen in those receiving the 'expensive' drug than in those who believed their treatment to be 'cheap' (Espay et al., 2015). These findings about the impact of 'prestige bias' on a technology's perceived effectiveness align with those of other studies, spanning both medical and other contexts (Díaz-Lago, Blanco and Matute, 2023).

NICE is therefore not alone in its inclination to give expensive innovations the benefit of the doubt. But in making such decisions, NICE increasingly commits itself to a path that may prove difficult to deviate from. Every technology recommended by NICE based on uncertain evidence or questionable cost-effectiveness sets a precedent that the influential pharmaceutical lobby will be eager for NICE to follow or build on in subsequent cases. Periodically, precedents set by individual cases may become codified and embedded in policy, making them even more difficult to challenge.[11] Once adopted into practice, technologies whose value is low or uncertain will often become the comparators against which new treatments are tested, building an increasingly unstable tower of recommendations in which the risk of decision-error – the unintentional adoption of a technology that is not clinically- or cost-effective – becomes increasingly likely. Such observations potentially cast NICE's high recommendation rate and support for innovation in a new light, as evidence of potentially harmful path dependency as well as the slow march of medical progress.

Conclusion: rearticulating NICE's values for the next 25 years

Norman Daniels has stated that 'there must be no secrets where justice is involved, for people should not be expected to accept decisions that affect their wellbeing unless they are aware of the grounds for those decisions', for people should not be expected to accept decisions that affect them if they cannot understand why they have been made (Daniels, 2000: 1301). Increasingly, NICE's decisions appear to be grounded not on its traditional values of fairness and reasonableness, but on its belief in the value of innovation and the ability of novel technologies to deliver societal benefits despite their associated uncertainties and opportunity cost.

If faced with explicitly explaining this shift in approach, NICE would likely characterise it as an example of values-improvement; a reflection of the rapidly changing world that we now live in and the potential role that innovation can play in fulfilling our healthcare needs. But NICE, to date, has been reluctant to acknowledge and justify this change, choosing instead to emphasise the purported continuity of its approach. While the Government has admitted that its concern for innovation is motivated by both the UK's health and its wealth (HM Government, 2021), NICE outwardly maintains that its concern for innovation is driven by the former; that its role remains to 'improve health and wellbeing

---

11 As in the formalisation of the £50,000/QALY threshold for end-of-life drugs. While the end-of-life criteria have since been replaced by a new severity modifier (Charlton, 2023), the specification of this standard has continued to be informed by the £50,000/QALY figure that emerged from practice.

by putting science and evidence at the heart of [. . .] decision-making' and that its decisions continue to be based on 'an assessment of population benefits and value for money' (NICE, 2020d; NICE, 2021b). In the words of NICE's Chief Executive, Dr Sam Roberts, and its Chairman, Sharmila Nebhrajani, NICE's 'core purpose is unchanged' – to drive 'efficient, informed decision-making' and to 'recommend only the most cost-effective treatments and procedures' (NICE, 2022b: 8–9).

In reality, NICE's core purpose does appear to have changed, from that of keeping potentially low value products out of the NHS, to actively facilitating the uptake of innovation. And in attempting to reconcile this new role with its old approach, NICE has found it necessary to stretch the definition of cost-effectiveness to its limit. This reluctance to fully acknowledge the new values driving decision-making is understandable: continuing to publicly subscribe to an approach based on reasonableness and fairness while acting in a way that also recognises other priorities is a sensible survival strategy for a body that relies on both public and political support for its existence. It may even be that such an approach can be defended as morally legitimate, on the grounds, for example, that it is supported by a democratically elected government. But in failing to fully acknowledge and justify how and why its approach has changed, NICE risks misleading those on whose behalf it acts.

The occasion of its 25th anniversary provides NICE with an opportunity to further reflect on and articulate its values and perhaps find a middle ground between what is politically necessary and what can be morally defended. In doing so, it is hoped that NICE can renew its moral mandate to set healthcare priorities on society's behalf and, in doing so, secure its future for another 25 years.

References

Atkinson, P. and Sheard, S. (2020) *Origins and Establishment of NICE (c. 1997–2002)*, Witness Seminar held online on 18 June 2020. University of Liverpool: Department of Public Health and Policy. Available at: https://www.liverpool.ac.uk/population-health-sciences/departments/public-health-and-policy/research-themes/governance-of-health/witness-seminars/ (Accessed 12 March 2023).

Bell, J. (2017) *Life Sciences Industrial Strategy: A Report to the Government from the Life Sciences Sector.* Available at: https://assets.publishing.service.gov.uk/govern ment/uploads/system/uploads/attachment_data/file/650447/LifeSciencesIndustrial Strategy_acc2.pdf (Accessed 9 March 2023).

Bullement, A., Taylor, M., McMordie, S.T., Waters, E. and Hatswell, A.J. (2019) 'NICE, in Confidence: An Assessment of Redaction to Obscure Confidential Information in Single Technology Appraisals by the National Institute for Health and Care Excellence', *PharmacoEconomics,* 37(11), pp.1383–90.

Cabinet Office (1999) *Modernising Government.* Cm 4310. London: The Stationery Office.

Chalkidou, K. (2012) 'Evidence and values: paying for end-of-life drugs in the British NHS', *Health Economics, Policy and Law*, 7(4), pp.393–409.

Charlton, V. (2020) 'NICE and fair? Health Technology Assessment policy under the UK's National Institute for Health and Care Excellence, 1999–2018', *Health Care Analysis*, 28(3), pp.193–227.

Charlton, V. (2022a) 'Does NICE apply the rule of rescue in its approach to highly specialised technologies?' *Journal of Medical Ethics*, 48, pp.118–25.

Charlton, V. (2022b) 'The normative grounds for NICE decision-making: a narrative cross-disciplinary review of empirical studies', *Health Economics, Policy and Law*, 17(4), pp.444–70.

Charlton, V. (2023) 'All health is not equal: the use of modifiers in NICE technology appraisal', *BMJ Evidence-Based Medicine*, 28, pp.247–50.

Charlton, V. and DiStefano, M. (2024) 'An empirical ethics study of the coherence of NICE technology appraisal policy and its implications for moral justification'. *BMC Medical Ethics* 25, 28. Available at: https://doi.org/10.1186/s12910-024-01016-0 (Accessed 22 April 2024).

Charlton, V. and Rid, A. (2019) 'Innovation as a value in healthcare priority-setting: the UK experience', *Social Justice Research*, 32, pp.208–38.

Claxton, K. and Culyer, A.J. (2006) 'Wickedness or folly? The ethics of NICE's decisions', *Journal of Medical Ethics*, 32, pp.373–77.

Claxton, K. and Culyer, A.J. (2007) 'Rights, responsibilities and NICE: a rejoinder to Harris', *Journal of Medical Ethics*, 33, pp.462–64.

Claxton, K. and Culyer, A.J. (2008) 'Not a NICE fallacy: a reply to Dr Quigley', *Journal of Medical Ethics*, 34, pp.598–601.

Clinicaltrials.gov. (2017) *A Phase III, Multicenter, Randomized, Placebo-Controlled Study of Atezolizumab in Combination with Nab-Paclitaxel Compared with Placebo with Nab-Paclitaxel for Participants with Previously Untreated Metastatic Triple-Negative Breast Cancer (IMpassion130): Statistical Analysis Plan*. Available at: https://www.clinicaltrials.gov/ProvidedDocs/91/NCT02425891/SAP_001.pdf (Accessed 30 March 2023).

Collins, M. and Latimer, N. (2013) 'NICE's end of life decision-making scheme: Impact on population health', *British Medical Journal*, 346:f1363.

Cookson, R. (2013) 'Can the NICE "end-of-life premium" be given a coherent ethical justification?', *Journal of Health Politics, Policy and Law*, 38(6), pp.1129–48.

Cookson, R., McDaid, D. and Maynard, A. (2001) 'Wrong SIGN, NICE mess: is national guidance distorting allocation of resources?': *British Medical Journal*, 323, pp.743–5.

Crinson, I. (2004) 'The politics of regulation within the "modernized" NHS: The case of beta interferon and the "cost-effective" treatment of multiple sclerosis', *Critical Social Policy*, 24(1), pp.30–49.

Daniels, N. (2000) 'Accountability for reasonableness', *British Medical Journal*, 321, pp.1300–01.

Daniels, N. and Sabin, J. (1997) 'Limits to Health care: fair procedures, democratic deliberation, and the legitimacy problem for insurers', *Philosophy & Public Affairs*, 26(4), pp.303–50.

Daniels, N. and Sabin, J. (2008) 'Accountability for reasonableness: an update', *British Medical Journal*, 337:a1850.

Davies, C., Barnett, E. and Wetherell, M. (2006). *Citizens at the Centre: Deliberative Participation in Healthcare Decisions*. Bristol: Policy Press.

Davis, C. and Abraham, J. (2013) *Unhealthy Pharmaceutical Regulation. Innovation, Politics and Promissory Science*. Basingstoke: Palgrave Macmillan.

Department for Business, Innovation and Skills (2011) *Strategy for UK Life Sciences*. London: Department for Business, Innovation and Skills.

Department of Health (1997) *The New NHS Modern, Dependable.* Cm 3807, London: The Stationery Office.

Department of Health (1998) *A First Class Service: Quality in the NHS.* London: Department of Health.

Department of Health (2009) *Innovation Pass Pilot: A Consultation on Proposals for an Innovation Pass Pilot.* London: Department of Health.

Department of Health and ABPI (2013) *2014 PPRS: Heads of Agreement.* London: Department of Health and ABPI.

Díaz-Lago, M., Blanco, F. and Matuter, H. (2023) 'Expensive seems better: the price of a non-effective drug modulates its perceived efficacy', *Cognitive Research: Principles and Implications,* 8(8).

Espay, A.J., Norris, M.M., Eliassen, J.C., Dwivedi, A., Smith, M.S., Banks, C., Allendorfer, J.B., Lang, A.E., et al. (2015) 'Placebo effect of medication cost in Parkinson disease', *Neurology,* 84(8), pp.794–802.

European Medicines Agency (2019) *Assessment Report: Tecentriq,* EMA/CHMP/425313/2019. Available at: https://www.ema.europa.eu/en/documents/variation-report/tecentriq-h-c-004143-x-0017-epar-assessment-report-extension_en.pdf (Accessed 30 March 2023).

European Medicines Agency (2023) *European Public Assessment Report: Tecentriq.* Available at: https://www.ema.europa.eu/en/medicines/human/EPAR/tecentriq (Accessed 30 March 2023)

Fleck, L.M. (2018) 'Controlling healthcare costs: just cost effectiveness or "just" cost effectiveness', *Cambridge Quarterly of Healthcare Ethics,* 27(2), pp.271–83.

Ford, A. (2015) 'Accountability for reasonableness: the relevance, or not, of exceptionality in resource allocation', *Medicine Health Care and Philosophy,* 18(2), pp.217–27.

Friedman, A. (2008) 'Beyond accountability for reasonableness', *Bioethics,* 22(2), pp.101–12.

Godin, B. (2016) 'Making sense of innovation: from weapon to instrument to buzzword', *Quaderni. Communication, technologies, pouvoir,* 90: pp.21–40.

Harris, J. (2005a) 'It's not NICE to discriminate', *Journal of Medical Ethics,* 31, p.373.

Harris, J. (2005b) 'Nice and not so nice', *Journal of Medical Ethics,* 31, pp.685–88.

Harris, J. (2006) NICE is not cost effective', *Journal of Medical Ethics,* 32, pp.378–80.

Harris, J. (2007) 'NICE rejoinder', *Journal of Medical Ethics,* 33, p.467.

HC Debate (1999) 'National Institute for Clinical Excellence (Amendment) Regulations 1999' (2 December).

Hickey, T. (2022) 'Legitimacy—*not Justice*—and the Case for Judicial Review', *Oxford Journal of Legal Studies,* 42(3), pp.893–917.

HM Government (2021) *Life Sciences Vision.* Available at: https://www.gov.uk/government/publications/life-sciences-vision (Accessed 25 March 2023).

Hofmann, B. (2002) 'Is there a technological imperative in health care?', *International Journal of Technology Assessment in Health Care,* 18 (3), pp.675–89.

Hong, Z. (2022) 'The population dynamics of the placebo effect and its role in the evolution of medical technology', *Human Ecology,* 50, pp.11–22.

Kennedy, I. (2009) *Appraising the Value of Innovation and other Benefits. A Short Study for NICE.* London: NICE.

King's Fund (2005) *An independent Audit of the NHS under Labour (1997–2005).* Available at: https://www.kingsfund.org.uk/sites/default/files/field/field_publication_file/independent-audit-nhs-under-labour-1997%E2%80%932005-sunday-times-march-2005.pdf (Accessed 18 March 2023).

Labour Party (1997) *New Labour Because Britain Deserves Better.* London: Labour Party.

Lauridsen, S. and Lippert-Rasmussen, K. (2009) 'Legitimate Allocation of Public Healthcare: Beyond Accountability for Reasonableness', *Public Health Ethics*, 2(1), pp.59–69.

Martin, S., Lomas, J., Claxton, K. and Longo, F. (2021) 'How effective is marginal healthcare expenditure? New evidence from England for 2003/04 to 2012/13', *Applied Health Economics and Health Policy*, 19, pp.885–903.

Maynard, A., Bloor, K. and Freemantle, N. (2004) 'Challenges for the National Institute for Clinical Excellence', *British Medical Journal*, 329, 227–29.

Miles, D., Gligorov, J., André, F., Cameron, D., Schneeweiss, A., Barrios, C., Xu, B., Wardley, A. et al. (2021) 'Primary results from IMpassion131, a double-blind, placebo-controlled, randomised phase III trial of first-line paclitaxel with or without atezolizumab for unresectable locally advanced/metastatic triple-negative breast cancer', *Annals of Oncology*, 32(8), pp.994–1004.

Nat. Biotechnol. (2009) 'A blueprint for biotech's blues' *Nature Biotechnology*, 27, p.675.

NHGRI (National Human Genome Research Institute) (2022) *Human Genome Project Timeline*. Available at: https://www.genome.gov/human-genome-project/timeline (Accessed 30 March 2023).

NICE (1999) *Framework Document*. London: NICE.

NICE (2004) *Guide to the Methods of Technology Appraisal*. London: NICE.

NICE (2005) *Social Value Judgements*. London: NICE.

NICE (2008) *Social Value Judgements*. 2nd edn. London: NICE.

NICE (2009) *Appraising Life-extending, End of Life Treatments*. London: NICE.

NICE (2013) *Guide to the Methods of Technology Appraisal*. PMG9. London: NICE.

NICE (2017) *NICE and the Life Sciences Industries*. Available at: https://www.nice.org.uk/Media/Default/News/NICE-and-the-life-sciences-industry.pdf (Accessed 30 March 2023).

NICE (2019) Appraisal Consultation Document: *Atezolizumab with nab-paclitaxel for treating PD-L1-positive, triple-negative, advanced breast cancer*. Available at: https://www.nice.org.uk/guidance/ta639/documents/129 (Accessed 20 March 2023).

NICE (2020a) Final Appraisal Determination: *Atezolizumab with nab-paclitaxel for untreated PD-L1-positive, locally advanced or metastatic, triple-negative breast cancer*. TA639.

NICE (2020b) *Glossary: Social Value Judgements*. Available at: https://www.nice.org.uk/glossary?letter=s (Accessed 20 October 2023).

NICE (2020c) 'Improved deal means new treatment for a type of advanced breast cancer can be recommended by NICE' (22 May). Available at: https://www.nice.org.uk/news/article/improved-deal-means-new-treatment-for-a-type-of-advanced-breast-cancer-can-be-recommended-by-nice (Accessed 25 March 2023).

NICE (2020d) *Our Principles: The Principles that Guide the Development of NICE Guidance and Standards*. London: NICE.

NICE (2021a) *NICE Strategy 2021 to 2026*. London: NICE.

NICE(2021b) *Our Charter*. Available at: https://www.nice.org.uk/about/who-we-are/our-charter (Accessed 21 March 2023).

NICE (2022a) 'Draft NICE guidance recommends innovative technology used to establish whether breast cancer has spread' (17 May). Available at: https://www.nice.org.uk/news/article/draft-nice-guidance-recommends-innovative-technology-used-to-establish-whether-breast-cancer-has-spread. (Accessed 25 March 2023).

NICE (2022b) *Annual Report and Accounts 2021/22*. London: NICE.

NICE (2022c) 'New life-extending treatment for rare forms of advanced gastroesophageal cancer recommended by NICE' (24 November). Available at: https://www.nice.

org.uk/news/article/new-life-extending-treatment-for-rare-forms-of-advanced-gas troesophageal-cancer-recommended-by-nice (Accessed 21 March 2023).

NICE (2022d) *NICE Health Technology Evaluations: The Manual*. PMG36. London: NICE.

NICE (2022e) 'NICE publishes new combined methods and processes manual and topic selection manual for its health technology evaluation programmes' (31 January). Available at: https://www.nice.org.uk/news/article/nice-publishes-new-combined-methods-and-processes-manual-and-topic-selection-manual-for-its-health-technol ogy-evaluation-programmes (Accessed 25 March 2023).

NICE (2022f) 'NICE recommends Enhertu for more people with advanced breast cancer' (20 December). Available at: https://www.nice.org.uk/news/article/nice-recom mends-enhertu-for-more-people-with-advanced-breast-cancer (Accessed 25 March 2023).

NICE (2022g) 'NICE recommends potentially life-changing treatment for people with short bowel syndrome' (1 June). Available at: https://www.nice.org.uk/news/article/ nice-recommends-potentially-life-changing-treatment-for-people-with-short-bowel-syndrome (Accessed 30 March 2023).

NICE (2022h) 'Over 700 people a year could benefit from a new potentially life-extending lung cancer drug which targets a specific genetic mutation' (14 April). Available at: https://www.nice.org.uk/News/Article/over-700-people-a-year-could-benefit-from-a-new-potentially-life-extending-lung-cancer-drug-which-targets-a-specific-genetic-mutation (Accessed 25 March 2023).

NICE (2022i) 'Targeted treatment for rare form of aggressive lung cancer gets NICE approval' (16 November). Available at: https://www.nice.org.uk/news/article/targeted-treatment-for-rare-form-of-aggressive-lung-cancer-gets-nice-approval (Accessed 25 March 2023).

NICE (2023a) *Managed Access*. Available at: https://www.nice.org.uk/about/what-we-do/our-programmes/managed-access (Accessed 18 March 2023).

NICE (2023b) 'More than 400 people set to benefit after NICE approves ground-breaking CAR-T therapy to treat aggressive form of blood cancer' (26 January). Available at: https://www.nice.org.uk/news/article/more-than-400-people-set-to-benefit-after-nice-approves-ground-breaking-car-t-therapy-to-treat-aggressive-form-of-blood-cancer (Accessed 25 March 2023).

NICE Citizens Council (2004) *Ultra Orphan Drugs*. London: NICE.

NICE Citizens Council (2008a) *Departing from the Threshold*. London: NICE.

NICE Citizens Council (2008b) *Quality Adjusted Life Years (QALYs) and Severity of Illness*. London: NICE.

NICE Citizens Council (2009) *Health Innovation and Value*. London: NICE.

NICE/NHS England (2022) *The Innovative Medicines Fund: Principles*. Available at: https://www.england.nhs.uk/wp-content/uploads/2022/06/B1686-the-innovate-medi cines-fund-principles-june-2022.pdf (Accessed 25 March 2023).

O'Mahony, J.F. and Paulden, M. (2014) NICE's selective application of differential discounting: ambiguous, inconsistent, and unjustified' *Value in Health*, 17(5), pp.493–96.

Osborne, S.P. and Brown, L. (2011) 'Innovation, public policy and public services delivery in the UK. The word that would be king?, *Public Administration*, 89(4), pp.1335–50.

Park, C. (2007) 'Technological Imperative', in Park, C., *A Dictionary of Environment and Conservation*. Oxford: Oxford University Press.

Paulden, M., O'Mahony, J.F., Culyer, A.J. and McCabe, C. (2014) 'Some inconsistencies in NICE's consideration of social values', *PharmacoEconomics*, 32, pp.1043–53.

Pearson, S.D. and Rawlins, M. (2005) 'Quality, innovation, and value for money: NICE and the British National Health Service', *Journal of the American Medical Association*, 294(20), pp.2618–22.

PMLive (2009) 'Government creates Office for Life Sciences' *PMLive* (6 April). Available at: https://www.pmlive.com/pharma_news/government_creates_office_for_life_sciences_141216 (Accessed 30 March 2023).

Office for Life Sciences (2018) *Industrial Strategy: Life Sciences Sector Deal 2*. Available at: https://www.gov.uk/government/publications/life-sciences-sector-deal/life-sciences-sector-deal-2-2018 (Accessed: 25 March 2023).

Quigley, M. (2007) 'A NICE fallacy', *Journal of Medical Ethics*, 33, p.465.

Rand, L. (2016). *Legitimate Priority-Setting: Refining Accountability for Reasonableness and its Application within NICE.* D.Phil. thesis, University of Oxford.

Rawlins, M. (2005) 'Pharmacopolitics and deliberative democracy', *Clinical Medicine*, 5(5), pp.471–75.

Rawlins, M. and Culyer, A.J. (2004) 'National Institute for Clinical Excellence and its value judgments', *British Medical Journal*, 329, pp.224–27.

Rawlins, M. and Dillon, A. (2005) 'NICE discrimination', *Journal of Medical Ethics*, 31, pp.683–84.

Richards, M. (2008) *Improving Access to Medicines for NHS Patients*. London: The Stationery Office.

Rid, A. (2009) 'Justice and procedure: how does 'accountability for reasonableness' result in fair limit-setting decisions?', *Journal of Medical Ethics*, 35, pp.12–16.

Rodwin, M.A. (2021) 'How the United Kingdom controls pharmaceutical prices and spending: learning from its experience' *International Journal of Health Services*, 51(2), pp.229–37.

Rumbold, B., Weale, A., Rid, A., Wilson, J. and Littlejohns, P. (2017) 'Public reasoning and health-care priority setting: the case of NICE', *Kennedy Institute of Ethics Journal*, 27(1), pp.107–34.

Schlander, M. (2008) 'The use of cost-effectiveness by the National Institute for Health and Clinical Excellence (NICE): no(t yet an) exemplar of a deliberative process', *Journal of Medical Ethics*, 34, pp.534–39.

Schmid, P., Adams, S., Rugo, H.S., Schneeweiss, A., Barrios, C.H., Iwata, H., Diéras, V., Hegg, R., et al. (2018) 'Atezolizumab and nab-paclitaxel in advanced triple-negative breast cancer', *New England Journal of Medicine*, 379, pp.2108–21.

Shah, K.K., Cookson, R., Culyer, A.J. and Littlejohns, P. (2013) 'NICE's social value judgements about equity in health and health care', *Health Economics Policy and Law*, 8(2), pp.145–65.

Smith, R. (2000) 'The failings of NICE: time to start work on version 2', *British Medical Journal*, 321(7273), pp.1363–64.

Stevens, A., Doyle, N., Littlejohns, P. and Docherty, M. (2012) 'National Institute for Health and Clinical Excellence appraisal and ageism', *Journal of Medical Ethics*, 38, pp.258–62.

Syrett, K. (2003) 'A technocratic fix to the "legitimacy problem"? The Blair government and health care rationing in the United Kingdom', *Journal of Health Politics, Policy and Law*, 28(4), pp.715–46.

Taylor, H. and Bell, J. (2016) *Accelerated Access Review: Final Report*. Available at: https://assets.publishing.service.gov.uk/media/5a7f3ca440f0b6230268e470/AAR_final.pdf (Accessed 21 March 2023).

Timmins, N., Rawlins, M. and Appleby, J. (2016) *A Terrible Beauty: A Short History of NICE*. Thailand: Health Intervention and Technology Assessment Programme.

Tymstra, T. (1989) 'The imperative character of medical technology and the meaning of 'anticipated decision regret'', *International Journal of Technology Assessment in Health Care*, 5(2), pp.207–13.

Van Wambeke, S. and Gyawali, B. (2021) Atezolizumab in Metastatic Triple-Negative Breast Cancer-No Contradiction in the Eyes of a Dispassionate Observer. *JAMA Oncol.*, 7(9), pp.1285–86.

Wanless, D. (2002) *Securing our Future Health: Taking a Long-term View – Final Report.* London: HM Treasury.

Wolf, S. and Berle, B.B. (1981) 'Meeting the challenge — summary and formulation', in Wolf, S. and Berle, B.B. (eds) *The Technological Imperative in Medicine: Proceedings of a Totts Gap Colloquium held June 15–17, 1980 at Totts Gap Medical Research Laboratories, Bangor, Pennsylvania.* Boston, MA: Springer US, pp.125–36.

6 Do NICE's HTA processes still lead to net improvements in NHS services?

James Wilson

Introduction

NICE's health technology appraisal (HTA) processes were introduced to improve the overall running of the NHS by reducing postcode prescribing, bringing a greater degree of cost control, and taking specific decisions about which drugs to fund out of the hands of politicians. Since 2010, NHS budgets have not kept pace with rising healthcare needs, leading among other effects to record waiting times for routine surgery. Over the same period, NICE has increasingly focused on promoting innovation and has given less weight within its deliberations to the opportunity costs of recommending cost-ineffective interventions. Thus, as budgets have become tighter within the NHS as a whole, NICE has been increasingly willing to recommend health technologies that are of relatively low cost-effectiveness, so long as they are innovative.

NICE's greater emphasis on innovation has effects that are on average negative for population health. However, a good health and care system will have goals beyond the maximisation of health, so a mean loss in population health would not automatically imply that the shift has been a net worsening for the NHS as a whole. Nonetheless, absent a plausible account of why it is ethically better to displace more health benefits than are created by prioritising innovation, it would be difficult to avoid the conclusion that this policy shift has contributed to a worsening of the care provided in the NHS. Unfortunately, NICE has not articulated such a rationale in detail. This chapter analyses NICE's approach to innovation, and to highly specialised technologies, arguing that even a sympathetic reconstruction of NICE's approach fails to uncover a convincing and consistent ethical framework. It is far from clear that NICE's current HTA processes lead to net improvements in NHS services.

The context

Section 233 of the Health and Social Care Act 2012 requires that in exercising its functions, NICE must have regard to three considerations. First, 'the broad

DOI: 10.4324/9781003501268-6

balance between the benefits and costs of the provision of health services or of social care', second 'the degree of need of persons for health services or social care in England', and third, 'the desirability of promoting innovation in the provision of health services or of social care in England'. The relationship between the benefits and costs of interventions delivered, and the degree of need for health and social care services have obvious – though contrasting – relationships to questions of fairness and equity in the delivery of services. I shall consider innovation shortly.

Focusing on the broad balance between benefits and costs requires above all, examining whether making a change such as introducing a new intervention, or revising guidance on management of a particular disease, would bring an overall improvement, or an overall worsening in the provision of health services or social care. The initial years of NICE coincided with an unprecedented rate of increase in the overall NHS budget, but since 2010 increases in health budgets have not kept pace with the rising costs of meeting health care needs. What counts as an overall improvement (or at least not worsening) needs to be understood against this background of rising scarcity within the health and social care system.

Waiting times, and a range of other service quality indicators, had been worsening significantly even before the Covid-19 pandemic. The diversion of healthcare resources away from non-Covid treatments exacerbated these problems in 2020–21, but performance against a range of indicators continued to decline once the pandemic subsided (Morris and Reed, 2022). Waiting lists for elective operations were larger by 2023 than at any point in the NHS's history, which was combined with a crisis in adult social care (Schlepper and Dodsworth, 2023). The health and care system as a whole has failed to scale its ability to meet health and social care needs to match increases in levels of these needs – and in some cases the absolute level of system capacity has declined, for example in numbers of GPs (BMA, 2023).

Under these circumstances, considering opportunity costs – those benefits that are already being provided that would be displaced by the introduction of new interventions – is of even greater importance than at NICE's inception. The simplest way to assess opportunity costs would be via a single measurement of value, such as a Quality Adjusted Life Year (QALY). On this simple view, both the QALYs to be gained, and those that would be displaced should be compared, and the intervention introduced only if the expectation would be that the benefits created would be greater than those displaced.

However, NICE's evaluative second requirement, namely to consider the *need* of persons for health services or social care, provides reasons for thinking that NICE would be failing to deliver on its role as set down in statute, if it focused only on the maximisation of QALYs in considering opportunity costs. In particular, needs that are urgent and important, such as providing intensive care unit treatment, can be costly to meet, as are drugs for very rare conditions.

It is very plausible to think that QALYs would be maximised in ways that require diverting resources from such relatively cost-ineffective measures to ones that create additional health benefits more cheaply (for example, public health preventive measures: see Chapter 7.) Nonetheless, the presumption that meeting health needs has an ethical importance that is separate from, and not reducible to maximising health benefits has a wide appeal: many worry that shifting resources from cost-ineffective treatment to more cost-effective prevention would *not* constitute an overall improvement in the health system, even though it would improve population health.[1]

In short, there should be no doubt that creating entitlements to novel interventions that are significantly less cost-effective than the mean cost-effectiveness of interventions within the health and social care system will tend to reduce, rather than increase, the overall health benefits the system generates. However, if QALY maximisation is an implausible goal for a health system, this loss of potential QALYs may yet be associated with an overall improvement rather than a worsening. This suggests that our conception of opportunity costs needs to shift in one of two ways. Either opportunity cost is just one of a number of ethically relevant concerns – such that, as in the case of funding intensive treatment units, it may be not just ethically permissible to pursue a policy that leads to more health being displaced than is created, but arguably ethically required to do so. Or alternatively, a broader vision of what counts as an opportunity cost could be adopted, such that we think of the opportunity costs of particular interventions in terms of the displacement of *value*, rather than health. On the broader view, opportunity costs map onto an account of whatever counts as an improvement for a health system, rather than presupposing that it is only the maximisation of health that matters. I suggest the latter is a more perspicuous framing of opportunity costs, as it foregrounds the crucial decisions in prioritisation, which is how to weigh the maximisation of health against other desiderata for a health system.

What counts as an improvement?

I use the concept of health system improvement to refer to the processes by which policymakers aim to deliver the best health system possible, given financial, broader resources, and other constraints (Wilson, 2023). I construe improvement in a deliberately broad and inclusive way, with the intention that it will be uncontentious (indeed truistic) that policymakers should aim to

---

1 I argue in Chapter 7 of Wilson (2021), and in Wilson (2022), that while it is legitimate for a democratic deliberation process to give a strong preference for treatment over prevention, there is no necessity to do so. Considered in themselves, the ethical arguments advanced for preferring expensive treatments to cheaper prevention are far from compelling.

improve health systems. What will be contentious is the principles that should guide improvement, and what improvement will require in practice. Thus, while the concept of health system improvement serves to indicate neutrally a topic of enquiry, there will be a variety of competing conceptions of health system improvement.

Within health system improvement, we should distinguish between means-improvement and values-improvement. Means-improvement involves mapping the ways in which a system converts inputs into outputs, and examining whether these could be reconfigured to allow the system as a whole better to achieve the values it aims to instantiate and promote. So, for example much of NICE's Clinical Guidance would count as means-improvement – aiming at better aligning treatment and clinical processes with the existing body of evidence. Values-improvement involves specifying and reconciling the values that a system should instantiate and promote. NICE's historical use of its Citizens Council to provide advice and guidance in respect of particular ethical questions such as whether NICE should use the Rule of Rescue (NICE Citizens Council, 2004), would count as values-improvement.

Attempts at means-improvement always presuppose an account of values. Sometimes these values may be left unarticulated – perhaps because they are believed to be too obvious to be worth reflecting on – but the fact remains that values are presupposed in any attempt at means improvement. A set of changes to a health system will count a successful means-improvement only if it allows the system as a whole to move in the direction of its values, as articulated and reconciled through earlier processes of values-improvement. It also follows that what counts as successful means-improvement will also shift if the values as articulated in a process of values-improvement change.

I have described values-improvement as a process. Just as an attempted means-improvement may make a system worse, if for example, it reduces the ability to respond to patient need or makes the system more brittle, so attempts at values-improvement can also make a system worse. At a high level, a process of values-improvement fails if the revised set of values it leads to are worse than the values from which the revisions set out.

This raises an important question about how we determine what makes one set of values *better* than another, rather than just different? Obviously, this is a large question, but one thing that is paramount is the kind of story those leading the process are able to tell about *why* moving from the former set of values to a new one counts as an improvement. Things that can be appealed to are both features of the process, for example broad and deep inclusion of a wide range of relevant stakeholders within the process that leads to the value revisions, and substantive improvements in values, such as reduction in unfair exclusions, improved alignment with broader sets of values widely accepted elsewhere such as human rights standards, decreases in errors, or increase in capacity. Similarly, in criticising a set of values as a worsening, we could appeal to elements of process or substantive failures in the values. For example, Charlton, Lomas and Mitchell (2022) argue that the changes made to the way that social values are handled in NICE's Methods Manual in 2022 could be criticised on both procedural and substantive grounds, and if they are correct in this, the changes would amount to a values-worsening rather than a values-improvement.

Distinguishing means-improvement from values-improvement allows us to pose a set of questions about how NICE's role relates to the rest of the NHS. NICE has a job to do, and in performing its role it must have regard to the three considerations with which this chapter began. However, from a broader perspective, the crucial question is whether if NICE performs its health technology assessments (HTA) in line with these three considerations, this will lead to a means-improvement in the health and social care system as a whole.

NICE's statutory duty to promote innovation in the provision of health services has been interpreted by it in a way that would license paying a greater incremental cost for interventions that are held to be 'innovative' than would be proportionate to the health benefits they provide. One central ethical challenge for this interpretation, which NICE has failed to discharge, is explaining how and why giving innovation an independent weighting provides an improvement either to NICE's processes, or to the broader health and social care system. One important question is whether the rationale is that promoting innovation in this way is a good means to improve the health and social care system over the medium or long term (even if it leads to short-term losses), or whether the rationale lies in benefits outside the direct sphere of the health and social care system (for example, by supporting the life sciences industry in the UK). Whatever its rationale, installing innovation as a third priority within NICE has contributed to the NHS as a whole in England becoming *less* able to meet a variety of patient needs, and less capable of delivering good value for money than it was previously. That the rise in the importance of innovation has led to a reduction in the focus given to the other two goals is not seriously in doubt (Charlton and Rid, 2019). In other words, the increased focus on innovation as an end in itself has led to a deterioration in fairness and equity, as well as lost health throughout the system. And so, it would be plausible to think that the focus on innovation has led to an overall improvement only if a perspective is adopted that goes beyond what is best for meeting the health needs of patients.

Health technology assessments

NICE's aims at a high level for its health technology assessments (HTA) follow the three laid down in statute that were cited at the beginning of this chapter. The HTA process takes for granted that resources are limited, and not all the care that would provide health benefits will be affordable. Prioritisation is thus required, and the process of HTA allows recommendations to be determined as to whether a technology should be made available within the NHS. The chosen mechanism for doing this is to assess the incremental cost-effectiveness ratio (ICER) of interventions, with the intention that this, in association with a set of baselines and modifiers (which are different between a general process, and one for very rare diseases) can be used to determine whether to recommend an intervention.

HTA can be done piecemeal or systematically. If it is done systematically, it allows for a ranking of all interventions, and thus a value threshold for a particular budget. Culyer (2016) provides a helpful simple model for this:

1. Work out how cost-effective each intervention is in £ per QALY.
2. Order all the interventions in order of cost-effectiveness. (Culyer asks us to visualise this as ordering books from left-to-right on a bookshelf in order of height; where height would represent cost-effectiveness: see Chapter 4.)
3. In funding interventions, start by funding the most cost-effective, and keep moving to the right of the shelf until the money runs out.
4. If the budget limit changes, the cost-effectiveness threshold for which interventions can be afforded also changes – rising as the budget increases, and falling as the budget decreases.

Culyer's model presupposes that it is *health gain* as measured via QALYs that a health system should be aiming to maximise. As we have already discussed, both NICE's duties under statute (and broader concerns from ethical theory) push towards a more complex account of what counts as an improvement, and what counts as a worsening within the health and social care system as a whole.

Culyer's general point still stands if we relax the assumption that a systematic approach to HTA should aim at the maximisation of QALYs. When looked at more broadly, a systematic approach to HTA should allow for an ordinal ranking of technologies such that, by use of this ordinal ranking, it is possible to order technologies from better to worse in relationship to the criteria by which 'better' is defined for the particular health and care system. If such an ordering is performed, and technologies are funded in order of precedence according to this ranking function, then allocating the budget in this way will be guaranteed to generate at least as much value as any alternative method (at least in so far as the value generated by each intervention is determined atomically rather than relationally or holistically).[2]

2 I argue elsewhere that there are many circumstances in which the value generated by one technology or intervention is determined relationally or holistically rather than atomically. See Wilson (2023) for more on this point. However, I leave this argument on one side for the purposes of this chapter.

Whatever account of value is selected for a systematic approach to HTA, the same model needs to be applied *both* to new interventions *and* to any existing interventions that would be displaced by the new interventions. For example, if it is appropriate to allow severity to count as a modifier for the ICERs for new interventions assessed (thus allowing recommendations of interventions with higher ICERs where the condition ameliorated is severe), then any such modifier would also need to be applied in decisions about which interventions to allow to be displaced, even if the decision is only to allow implicit rationing by queuing (Wilson, 2023). Unless decisions about what to defund are also driven by the same process, then particularly where recommendations are made to fund interventions that are well above the mean cost of creating one QALY in the health system, such decisions are likely to displace more value than they create.

HTA is piecemeal, rather than systematic, if some but not all interventions are assessed. Where HTA is piecemeal, it does not allow for a complete ordinal ranking. As a result, on a piecemeal approach, it may not be immediately obvious whether, when new interventions are introduced as a result of the HTA process, and others displaced, this will in fact lead to an improvement rather than a worsening given the system's own stated goals.

The health and social care system of which NICE is part adopts a piecemeal rather than a systematic model of HTA. Some but not all novel interventions are assessed, and there are many interventions that have been in long use that have not received an HTA. Even those interventions that are assessed are not assessed in a way that would allow for a clear ordinal ranking between them: the HTA process delivers a result of either a recommended, optimised (recommended for a smaller group), only in research, or not recommended – and so it is better to see it as supporting a satisficing rather than a maximising approach to value (Rumbold et al., 2017).

While the approach taken makes an ordinal ranking of interventions impossible, it is possible to estimate the less statistically demanding figure of the mean cost of creating one QALY within the health system, which Claxton et al. (2015) calculated at a little under £13,000. If this is anything like correct, then it would obviously be the case that NICE's standard HTA process, which tends to wave through any interventions that deliver QALYs at under £20,000 per QALY, and also funds interventions at up to £50,000 per QALY where there are relevant factors such as severity, frequently allows new interventions that would be predicted to displace more health benefit than they create.

For the reasons already noted, even if such interventions tend to displace more health benefit than they create, this is not yet to say that they amount to overall worsenings rather than improvements of the health and care system. Nonetheless, given both the lack of systematic and rigorous processes for deprioritisation, and the extent of implicit rationing and rising waiting lists, there is no strong positive reason to think that the present net result of NICE HTA recommendations is an overall improvement to the health and social care system. As we shall shortly examine, Highly Specialised Technologies (HST) raise this problem even more strongly, given that they are funded at a baseline of £100,000 per incremental QALY and may reach up to £300,000 per incremental QALY.

The value of innovation

One way in which one might attempt to explain how NICE HTA recommendations *do* lead to improvements within the NHS even if they end up displacing more health benefits than they create is via the value of innovation. As we noted, there is a statutory duty on NICE to have regard to 'the desirability of promoting innovation in the provision of health services or of social care'. The fact that the duty is there implies that policymakers thought that there is *something* that would be improved if NICE had reference to this duty in conducting its affairs.

Nonetheless it is not obvious that it is conducive to overall improvement within the health and care system for HTA processes to place a premium on innovation, and thus treat the fact that an intervention is deemed 'innovative' to justify spending significantly more per incremental QALY on it than would be the case if it were not deemed to be 'innovative'.

As Charlton and Rid (2019) argue, while the Health and Social Care Act 2012 led to a significant increase in mentions of innovation within NICE's HTA processes, neither the intention of NICE's policy on innovation nor what counts as innovative, has ever been spelled out in detail. Charlton and Rid suggest that the most coherent reconstruction of NICE's policy is that an intervention is innovative only if the following three conditions apply: (a) the intervention is novel, (b) the treatment gives rise to significant or substantial health benefits (a 'step-change'), and (c) that the health benefit is not adequately captured in the ICER.

Charlton and Rid's account provides a plausible reconstruction of how the policy is intended to work, but as their own analysis underlines, if they are correct about the requirements of the policy, it would appear that the policy has often been misinterpreted by both NICE committees and applicants. On their analysis, there are significant inconsistencies in the way in which each of the three requirements has been interpreted by different committees, for example, the requirement that there should be a substantial benefit was sometimes interpreted in a way that almost any intervention would meet the bar and at other times in a stricter way (Charlton and Rid, 2019, p. 223). Whether there are benefits that are not fully captured in the QALY is something that HTA committees already need to consider in all cases; and so it is unclear what this requirement adds in theory, and as Charlton and Rid examine, in practice it has led to significant inconsistencies with some committees taking improving earning capacity of patients to be relevant while other committees rule this out (Charlton and Rid, 2019).

A more fundamental point is that, even if the policy as interpreted by Charlton and Rid were applied consistently, it would remain unclear why 'innovation' thus circumscribed should be rewarded. It is worth noting that the conception of innovation implicit within NICE's processes is inconsistent with that used within patent law. No invention is patentable unless it meets a test of novelty. NICE does not appraise generic drugs through its HTA processes, and the vast majority of interventions that NICE examines in HTA are pharmaceuticals that are under patent, so *all* these interventions have by definition already met a threshold of novelty. Thus, 'innovative' as used by NICE picks out a subset of those interventions that for the purposes of intellectual property law have been judged to be novel.

Patents on pharmaceuticals are not without ethical challenges (Wilson, 2012a), but there are good reasons for wanting to create incentive structures to encourage innovation through intellectual property law, and thereby make drug discovery attractive for businesses to invest in. However, given that such incentives for research and development are provided by intellectual property law, it is not immediately obvious why an additional policy of incentivisation would be required, which applies only once a new product has been brought to market.

Insofar as the presence of 'innovation' as defined by NICE allows higher prices to be paid than would otherwise be permitted, and the budget is limited, the greater the innovation premium or incentive, the greater the health losses will be elsewhere in the system. Even if these incentives are successful at bringing into use some innovative treatments that would otherwise have been excluded on grounds of poor value for money, and thereby benefit patients who can access the treatments, there is an obvious opportunity cost to other patients. Patients will not, on average, be benefited by an innovation premium, even if some are.

So the challenge in providing an ethical rationale for the innovation premium is to explain either why initial appearances are deceptive, and the innovation premium is in fact on average beneficial for patients, or why, despite not being on average beneficial for patients, the innovation premium nonetheless would be expected to bring an overall improvement.

One obvious defence of the innovation premium is to argue that it is only over the short-term that it appears to be on average harmful to patients. It could be argued to be a loss-leader: we pay now in order to make it possible for innovation to continue in the future and also because the innovations that are expensive now will become cheaper as they go off patent and become available as generics. On this line of thinking, paying more now is an investment in cheaper and more effective drugs in the future.

This is the general economic justification given for intellectual property law, but it works much better at a global level than it does as an argument about how England should spend its health budget. England is a relatively small percentage of the global market for pharmaceuticals (around 3%); and so it is clearly not the case that pharmaceutical innovation would be slowed significantly, were NICE *not* to incorporate an innovation premium in its HTA processes. If the NHS relied heavily on other health systems subsiding innovation, there might potentially be an argument to be made about the ethics of free-riding (Wilson, 2012b), though it is notable that such an argument has not been advanced as the rationale for NICE's focus on innovation. As a result, in so far as an innovation premium benefits patients in England, it may be best to think of it not as providing incentives for innovation per se, but rather incentives for manufacturers to license drugs in the UK and to engage with the NICE HTA process. The risk that the innovation premium attempts to forestall may not be that drug discovery will not take place at all, but that manufacturers (particularly in a post-Brexit world) may not take the UK market to be worth engaging with.

It is far from clear that adopting an innovation premium is, in fact, on average beneficial for users of the NHS in the short or medium term. Considered from the perspective of benefiting patients, it would be perverse to have an innovation premium unless there is reason to think that the interventions funded under this premium will in the medium term tend to become available at a price and value point that will not displace more value than they create. If the prices of interventions that were initially funded as 'innovative' remain high over the medium term, then adopting such interventions makes it harder for a health system to achieve its goals.

While arguments for thinking that an innovation premium will lead to improved average health are unconvincing, the loss of health gains that could be obtained more cheaply through adopting other priorities does not yet entail that the innovation premium makes the health and care system as a whole worse. There may be features of specific patient groups or specific healthcare needs that justify very high prices, even though this has opportunity costs for others. For example, it could be argued that innovative technologies deliver especially valuable health benefits. Or it could be argued that the benefits brought by innovative technologies are either not properly captured by NICE's standard HTA processes, or difficult to measure.

These kinds of arguments are most plausible in the case of interventions necessary to treat serious but very rare conditions, such as those funded under NICE's Highly Specialised Technologies (HST) programme. However, as the next section explores, the factors that make it ethically plausible to think that a health system should be willing to pay significantly more per QALY in such cases are not closely related to the level of innovation that an intervention shows.

The Highly Specialised Technologies Programme

As NICE makes clear in the Methods Manual, the HST programme is 'designed to be used in exceptional circumstances', namely very rare diseases that by their nature have small numbers of patients, and in addition have 'limited or no treatment options', and 'challenges for research and difficulties with collecting evidence, because of the uniqueness of the disease' (NICE, 2022, sec. 7.1.3). The Manual explains that the HST programme is required by fairness and equity: it aims to 'secure fairer and more equitable treatment access for very small populations with very rare diseases', and to 'recognise that an approach that maximises health gain for the NHS may not always be acceptable: it could deliver results that are not equitable' (NICE, 2022, sec. 7.1.4).

NICE's standard HTA process now (post 2022) is formalised in a way that the baseline ICER is £20,000 per QALY, which with the severity weighting can go out to an ICER of £50,000. The HST process has a baseline ICER of £100,000 per QALY, with the ability to go up to £300,000 per QALY. The Manual is frank that each time a HST is recommended, 'the NHS must commit to allocate resources that would have otherwise been used on activities that would be expected to generate greater health benefits' (NICE, 2022, sec. 7.1.5). It talks of the need to 'strike a balance between the desirability of supporting access to treatments for very rare diseases against the inevitable reduction in overall health gain across the NHS that this will cause' (NICE, 2022, sec. 7.1.5).

One means by which HST aims to strike the appropriate balance is to draw the eligibility criteria in a deliberately fairly narrow way: the processes 'intentionally do not seek to capture every case when there are challenges in generating an evidence base or when there is a small population with a rare disease' (NICE, 2022, sec. 7.1.5). Another is that HST processes are used only when a disease is *very* rare: orphan drug designations are available from the MHRA and the European Medicines Agency when the prevalence of a disease is no more than 5 in 10,000 people, but the NICE HST process only applies to diseases that have a prevalence that is 25 times smaller, at less than 1 in 50,000 people.

The HST programme thus clearly raises ethical questions, which are alluded to with the references to equity and the discussion of opportunity costs in the Manual, but these ethical questions are not faced head-on. This is odd, given that similar questions *were* taken up by the NICE Citizens Council when it examined ultra orphan drugs in 2004 and the rule of rescue in 2006, and as the next section examines, the Citizens Council's conclusions are not easy to reconcile with NICE's current approach.

The costs of drug development provide obvious reasons why drugs for orphan diseases tend to have higher ICERs than drugs for common diseases, and why drugs for ultra orphan diseases tend to have even higher ICERs. But it is nonetheless surprising from an ethical perspective to adopt the approach that NICE has by segmenting HTA into two separate processes with wildly different baseline ICER requirements, especially as the eligibility require-ments for HST only apply when the prevalence of a disease is 25 times lower than the threshold for an orphan drug designation. One implication of NICE's approach is that there are many diseases that are rare enough that ICERs for novel interventions are likely to be significantly higher than for more common diseases, but which will not be nearly rare enough to receive an HST designa-tion. Such cases of disease that are rare, but not rare enough for HST, include cystic fibrosis and Fragile X syndrome.

Clarke, Ellis and Brownrigg (2021) found that orphan drugs assessed via NICE's standard Single Technology Assessment (STA) seemed to suffer disad-vantages both relative to non-orphan drugs, and relative to those assessed via HST. As compared to non-orphan drugs, the assessment of orphan drugs took significantly longer within the STA process; and while the chance of receiving a positive recommendation was comparable between orphan and non-orphan drugs, the orphan drugs were meeting an unmet healthcare need. Relative to HST, chances of receiving a positive recommendation were lower and decisions took longer.

In short, NICE's current processes end up disadvantaging those with rare, but not very rare, diseases. And so, even if it is true that it would be unfair not to make special provision for very rare diseases, the way that this has been done risks creating other unfairnesses for groups of patients who have rare, but not very rare, diseases. We will now consider the question of the ethical status of rar-ity per se: does the rarity of a disease sometimes provide good reasons to adopt a different approach to HTA, in particular by shifting baseline ICERs?

Rarity and severity

If the rarity of disease is separated from all other features, and considered on its own, it is far from obvious that it matters ethically. McCabe (2005) asks us to imagine a case where all features are held the same between two diseases, except that one is ten times rarer and ten times less cost-effective to treat than the other: those with the rarer condition 'have the same personal characteristics, the same prognosis without treatment, and the same capacity to benefit from the treat-ments' (McCabe, 2005, p. 1018). If we are right to think that cost-effectiveness matters in the usual case, then other things being equal, we should prefer a health gain that is in all respects similar but ten times cheaper to one that is ten times as expensive. Indeed, if all else is equal, we should rank the one much more highly than the other, as the opportunity cost of treating one individual with the more expensive condition would be that ten individuals with the same prognosis and capacity to benefit would go untreated. Assuming the budget is limited, it might well be the case that the first should be funded for many patients, while the sec-ond will lose out and not be funded at all.

Thus, the ethical challenge posed by special provisions for very rare diseases is to explain why it is ethically better if a greater number of individuals are denied treatment in order to allow treatment for a smaller number with rarer conditions, even though the prognosis and capacity to benefit of individuals in both groups is the same. When put in such stark terms, it becomes clear that absent such a justification, paying a much higher ICER for very rare conditions is *unethical*.

When the NICE Citizens Council examined ultra orphan drugs in 2004, more than half thought that much higher ICERs should be paid for rare conditions, but those who did favour special arrangements tended to be sceptical that it was rarity itself that made the difference: 'people stressed that it was because these rare diseases are often so severe that it is justified. On its own, the rarity of a disease, would not give it special status' (NICE Citizens Council, 2004, p. 7).

NICE's standard HTA processes and HST both provide approaches (albeit different approaches) to responding to severity. The HST programme responds to the value of severity, in so far as the HST pathway is defined in such a way that technologies can be routed to it only if the condition that will be treated is severe. While there will be non-severe conditions that could be treated for very rare diseases, such interventions are out of scope for HST. NICE's standard HTA processes also include severity as a value: in the 2022 Methods Manual, severity is a value that justifies a modifier of up to 1.7x on the baseline cost-effectiveness ratios. The presence of severity as a value in both NICE's standard HTA and HST processes works to undermine the claim the HST programme is justified *because* rare diseases are severe.

If we step back a bit from NICE's actual processes, it is clear that the severity of a condition is orthogonal to its rarity. A condition can be common but very severe, as well as very rare but mild. There is no reason to think that the suffering caused by very rare conditions is per se *more severe* than for more common conditions, and so it is not obvious how giving due weight to the ethical importance of severity would justify different ICERs for rare conditions. There is thus no reason to think that severity provides an additional reason for giving extra weight to HST, over and above the ethical weight that would be due to severity in other cases. In so far as severity matters by itself, it is an argument to fund treatments for very severe conditions at a premium regardless of their rarity, rather than a consideration that would apply only to very rare conditions. So, even if severity matters intrinsically, this does not by itself provide an ethical justification for special processes for very rare diseases.

Bad luck and nonabandonment

While the fact that an ailment is rare does not per se make it more agonising or more deadly than one that is common, nonetheless there is a non-accidental relationship between the rarity of a disease and the low cost-effectiveness of the drugs needed to treat it. Even if, other things being equal, cheap health benefits should be ranked more highly than less cost-effective health benefits, and even if other things being equal, the fact that a condition is rare is not intrinsically ethically significant, we might still think that the combination of the two creates an ethical claim: if there is a non-accidental correlation between treatments that are available for rare conditions and expensive treatments.

There may be cases where the intersection of two factors has unfair implications, even if by themselves neither has this implication separately. This is sometimes explained via the idea of nonabandonment – the idea that everyone deserves or has a strong claim to some kind of effective treatment for their condition, even if it would be very expensive to provide it (Gericke, Busse and Riesberg, 2005). It might be argued that giving a significant weight to nonabandonment is a plausible way of interpreting the idea of treating citizens as equals in this context.

Luck egalitarians claim that it is unfair if someone is worse off than others through no fault of their own. It looks to be a matter of bad luck that any particular individual (a) develops a fatal or debilitating disease that they had no ability to affect, and it is a further piece of bad luck that (b) in virtue of its rarity, their disease is highly likely to be much more expensive to treat than a common disease. This might provide an argument for thinking that something like HST should be put into operation in order to counteract this bad luck. However, the idea of luck is itself somewhat nebulous and subject to different interpretations (Lippert-Rasmussen, 2023). While developing a fatal or debilitating disease that one had no ability to affect is often given as a paradigm case of bad luck, it is not immediately clear whether the badness of luck should be graded such that *very* bad luck creates a stronger claim to aid than ordinarily bad luck (and if so, by how much).

In addition, what counts as bad luck in the context of HTA decisions about which particular interventions to include within the scope of public funding is not easily separable from the policy decisions that are taken. As was discussed earlier, the HST programme NICE employs has a cut-off of 1 in 50,000. Given this decision, it would then seem to be a matter of bad lack for those individuals with a condition that is rare enough that is too expensive to be funded under the normal HTA rules, but not rare enough to benefit from the HST process. So while it might be the case that some special provision for rare diseases would follow from luck egalitarianism, it is not obvious that NICE's specific approach would be the best way of doing so.

Conclusion

NICE began with a remit to reduce postcode prescribing, bring a greater degree of cost control, and take specific decisions about which drugs to fund out of the hands of politicians. In its early years, NICE was able to stand up for the importance of cost-effectiveness analysis and consideration of opportunity costs in making decisions about when interventions should be recommended for use in the NHS, even while doing so would have been tricky for politicians. Both NICE and the broader NHS context have changed significantly since 2010. NHS budgets have failed to keep pace with rising healthcare needs, but during the same time period, NICE has de-emphasised the opportunity costs of recommending cost-ineffective interventions. The combined effect is that NICE recommendations are increasingly likely to lead to the displacement of more health benefits than they create, for example, leading to cuts to other services or degradation of service quality.

From an ethical perspective, the important question is whether there are reasons to think that the decreased salience given to opportunity costs has brought net ethical benefits despite being on average negative for population health. This chapter analysed NICE's approach to innovation, and to highly specialised technologies, arguing that even a sympathetic reconstruction of NICE's approach fails to uncover a convincing ethical justification for the policies currently adopted. While it is plausible to think that sometimes the benefits of a health technology are not well captured by the QALY, and that a health system should be willing to pay more per QALY for interventions that treat severe conditions, neither consideration is specific to innovative technologies. As Victoria Charlton examines in Chapter 5, the increased emphasis on innovation is most plausibly explained by a perceived need on NICE's part to align with the political priorities of the government's industrial strategy.

HST provides the most radical departure from a maximising approach, and here also there is much that is puzzling, or ethically questionable, about NICE's policy – from the eligibility requirements to the conception of fairness it draws upon. In both cases, what is striking is that while the processes as set out in the Methods Manual and realised in committee review have become ever more well-articulated and rigorous, the ethical framework within which these processes unfold has become sketchier. NICE itself seems to have retreated from the project of debating and publicly justifying the core values at the heart of its approach, just as those values have become more ethically questionable. It is much less clear than it was 25 years ago that NICE's health technology assessments lead to an overall improvement rather than worsening of the service that the NHS as a whole can provide.

References

BMA (2023) *Pressures in General Practice Data Analysis*. Available at: https://www. bma.org.uk/advice-and-support/nhs-delivery-and-workforce/pressures/pressures-in-general-practice-data-analysis (Accessed 10 May 2023).

Charlton, V. and Rid, A. (2019) 'Innovation as a value in healthcare priority-setting: the UK experience', *Social Justice Research*, 32(2), pp.208–38.

Charlton, V., Lomas, J. and Mitchell, P. (2022) 'NICE's new methods: putting innovation first, but at what cost?', *British Medical Journal*, 379, p.e071974.

Clarke, S., Ellis, M. and Brownrigg, J. (2021) 'The impact of rarity in NICE's health technology appraisals', *Orphanet Journal of Rare Diseases*, 16(1), p.218.

Claxton, K., Martin, S., Soares, M., Rice, N., Spackman, E., Hinde, S., Devlin, N., Smith, P.C., and Sculpher, M. (2015) 'Methods for the estimation of the National Institute for Health and Care Excellence cost-effectiveness threshold,' *Health Technology Assessment*, 19(14), pp.1–503.

Culyer, A.J. (2016) 'Cost-effectiveness thresholds in health care: a bookshelf guide to their meaning and use', *Health Economics, Policy and Law*, 11(4), pp.415–32.

Gericke, C.A., Busse, R. and Riesberg, A. (2005) 'Ethical issues in funding orphan drug research and development', *Journal of Medical Ethics*, 31(3), pp.164–68.

Lippert-Rasmussen, K. (2023) 'Justice and Bad Luck', in Zalta, E.N., and Nodelman, U. (eds) *The Stanford Encyclopedia of Philosophy*. Spring 2023. Metaphysics Research Lab, Stanford University. Available at: https://plato.stanford.edu/archives/spr2023/entries/justice-bad-luck/ (Accessed 8 May 2023).

McCabe, C. (2005) 'Orphan drugs and the NHS: should we value rarity?', *British Medical Journal*, 331(7523), pp.1016–19.

Morris, J. and Reed, S. (2022) *How Much is Covid-19 to Blame for Growing NHS Waiting Times?* London: Nuffield Trust. Available at: https://www.nuffieldtrust.org.uk/resource/how-much-is-covid-19-to-blame-for-growing-nhs-waiting-times (Accessed 22 April 2023).

NICE (2022) *NICE Health Technology Evaluation Topic Selection: The Manual*. London: NICE. Available at: https://www.nice.org.uk/process/pmg37/chapter/about-this-guide (Accessed 12 April 2023).

NICE Citizens Council (2004) *Ultra Orphan Drugs*. London: NICE.

Rumbold, B., Weale, A., Rid, A., Wilson, J., and Littlejohns, P. (2017) 'Public reasoning and health-care priority setting: the case of NICE', *Kennedy Institute of Ethics Journal*, 27(1), pp.107–34.

Schlepper, L. and Dodsworth, E. (2023) *The Decline of Publicly Funded Social Care for Older Adults*. London: Nuffield Trust and Health Foundation. Available at: https://www.nuffieldtrust.org.uk/resource/the-decline-of-publicly-funded-social-care-for-older-adults (Accessed 22 April 2023).

Wilson, J. (2012a) 'On the value of the intellectual commons', in Lever, A. (ed.) *New Frontiers in the Philosophy of Intellectual Property*. Cambridge: Cambridge University Press.

Wilson, J. (2012b) 'Paying for patented drugs is hard to justify: an argument about time discounting and medical need', *Journal of Applied Philosophy*, 29(3), pp.186–99.

Wilson, J. (2021) *Philosophy for Public Health and Public Policy: Beyond the Neglectful State*. Oxford: Oxford University Press.

Wilson, J. (2022) 'When does precision matter? Personalized medicine from the perspective of public health', in Barilan, Y.M., Brusa, M., and Ciechanover, A. (eds) *Can Precision Medicine Be Personal; Can Personalized Medicine Be Precise?* Oxford: Oxford University Press, pp.173–86.

Wilson, J. (2023) 'What makes a health system good? From cost-effectiveness analysis to ethical optimisation in health systems', *Medicine, Health Care and Philosophy*, 26, pp.351–65.

7 Public Health at NICE

Methods, politics and policy

Michael P. Kelly

Introduction

The methodological principles which NICE applied to produce public health guidelines were based on its experience of undertaking technology appraisals and developing clinical guidelines. The methods also drew heavily on work by the Health Development Agency (HDA), the Centre for Reviews and Dissemination in York, the EPPI-Centre (the Evidence for Policy and Practice Information and Co-ordinating Centre), the Cochrane Collaboration, and the health economics principles of cost utility analysis. The NICE approach to public health owed much to the Research and Development Strategy published by the Department of Health in 2001 (Department of Health, 2001). This chapter describes how these different strands came together, and the resulting scientific and political consequences. It will describe the methodological innovations which the work entailed. The practical problems associated with the development of the public health evidence base and its application will be outlined. The chapter will consider the ways in which, in addressing the structural determinants of health inequalities in evidence and guidelines, NICE found itself embroiled in various political storms. This occurred when the scientific evidence, and some of the public health evidence-based guidelines which NICE produced, did not align with prevailing government policies nor commercial orthodoxies. The tensions arising from working at the interface of scientific evidence, public health practice, policymaking and politics will be described with reference to specific guidelines.

The story in broad outline

This is a methodological story about the way that policy, science and politics became entwined in the development of public health guidelines at NICE. As proposed in the Research and Development Strategy of the Department of Health published in 2001 (Department of Health, 2001), a newly formed Arm's-Length Body – the Health Development Agency (HDA) – started applying, in the same

DOI: 10.4324/9781003501268-7

year, the principles of evidence-based medicine (EBM) to public health problems, with a particular focus on reducing health inequalities. Four years later in 2005, the HDA was amalgamated with NICE. NICE had at that point just acquired the responsibility to develop public health guidelines. In the new Centre for Public Health Excellence in NICE, the work on the application of EBM to public health and to develop guidelines was led by the team that had applied EBM to public health in the HDA. The team now had the additional responsibility for developing guidelines on cost-effective population health improvement and disease prevention. The focus on health inequalities was to be retained. Methodologically, public health at NICE then made considerable progress as it sought to embrace evidence from psychology, sociology, geography, political science and epidemiology, as well as clinical medicine. It also had to find a way to apply the methods of health economics, particularly cost utility analysis, to the world of preventive medicine (Kelly et al., 2005). This became one of the most systematic programmes designed to apply EBM to public health globally.

When NICE began working on public health guidelines the methods to embrace a wide discipline base and the traditional techniques of cost utility economic analysis to public health, were not well-developed. While the methods of Health Technology Assessment were becoming increasingly sophisticated, there had not been much systematic work on public health evidence-based guidelines in the UK, although the policy strategy to do so had been in place since 2001 (Department of Health, 2001). By 2005, HDA had developed methods to do public health evidence synthesis and review (Swann et al., 2005) and had published a series of Evidence Briefings summarising the state of the evidence base. The Centre for Reviews and Dissemination in York had likewise a programme of work concerned with evidence review in public health (NHS Centre for Reviews and Dissemination, 1995). There was some work in the USA, at the Centre for Disease Control in Atlanta (Zaza, Briss and Harris, 2005). But none of this was concerned with developing national public health practice or policy guidelines – the post-2005 role for NICE. It was to some extent, if not a blank canvas, then a very thinly populated landscape. There were no off-the-shelf scientific or methodological handbooks or protocols readily available. The scientific challenges NICE faced were considerable. The move to develop public health guidelines was a bold experiment and one that revealed in stark relief the ways in which evidence and politics can collide. It also showed how the well-honed methods of evidence-based medicine and Health Technology Appraisal did not fit easily onto the canvas of public health.

The origins of an idea

The idea in question is that of applying EBM to Public Health. But what is EBM, and where had it come from? A good starting point is the book *Effectiveness and Efficiency: Random Reflections on Health Services,* by Archie Cochrane, published in 1972 (Cochrane, 1972). Much of the way that EBM subsequently took shape was influenced by Cochrane's ideas. In his book, Cochrane asked a series of questions about clinical medicine, especially in the UK context. The questions were as follows. Do we know whether intervention x for problem y is effective? How do we know it is effective? How do we know whether it is more or less effective than intervention z? On what basis do we make that judgement of effectiveness? Do we know what it costs? Is it cost-effective? If it is not cost-effective, why is it being used? What are the dangers posed to patients of treatments about which we are scientifically uncertain? Are interventions dangerous? Why do we use potentially dangerous or worthless interventions?

Cochrane argued that evidence derived from properly conducted investigations, especially randomised controlled trials (RCTs), was the best way to answer these questions (Kelly, 2018). He also suggested the need for a system to monitor and systematically record trial results. However, it was not until some years later, in Canada, that the EBM idea really took off. David Sackett at McMaster University, and a group of collaborators, coined the term EBM. They stated 'Evidence-based medicine de-emphasizes intuition, unsystematic clinical experience, and pathophysiologic rationale as sufficient grounds for clinical decision-making and stresses the examination of evidence from clinical research' (The Evidence-Based Medicine Working Group, 1992: 2420). In 1996 Sackett and colleagues argued that EBM was 'the conscientious, explicit, and judicious use of current best evidence in making decisions about the care of individual patients. The practice of evidence-based medicine means integrating individual clinical expertise with the best available external clinical evidence from systematic research' (Sackett et al., 1996: 71). Gradually the idea that the RCT was the best method for determining clinical effectiveness took root and has since been widely adopted. It is now the standard method, often referred to as a gold standard, with syntheses of trial results as the best guide to the overall state of the evidence (Egger, Higgins and Davey Smith, 2022; Greenhalgh, 2001).

In 1993, the Cochrane Collaboration had been established, taking its name from Archie Cochrane. It was the crystallisation of his suggestion that there should be a system for making available systematic reviews of all relevant RCTs of health care (Kelly, 2018). The idea was that the review, appraisal and synthesis of the results of the trials should be conducted to the highest standards. Another important principle was that negative results should also be published to avoid the intrinsic positive publication bias in the evidence base (Chalmers, Dickersin and Chalmers, 1992). The existence of the Cochrane Collaboration has been a major pillar in the development of EBM and evidence-based public health, and it is a resource widely used by researchers, guideline developers, methodologists, public health practitioners and clinicians worldwide.

It was against this scientific background that NICE came into existence in 1999. It was to conduct appraisals of new pharmaceuticals to ascertain whether they were good value for money for the NHS. Soon afterwards NICE began developing clinical guidelines. NICE was important because it became the most high-profile public body in the UK practicing EBM as the basis for its decisions.

While work was getting underway in NICE with its focus on clinical medicine, the idea that public health should likewise get in on the EBM act, was gaining ground (Department of Health, 2001). It was acknowledged that there were considerable deficiencies in the generation and use of evidence in public health in the UK. Sir John Pattison, then Director of Research and Development at the Department of Health, indicated that there was a need to 'extend the evidence base, and to improve the use of the knowledge that we already have' (Department of Health, 2001: foreword). The Department of Health set out a strategy for health improvement, focussing on population health and reducing health inequalities (Department of Health, 2001). It noted that a range of organisations like the Research Councils and Government Departments had a role to play. The document identified a need for syntheses and summaries of the evidence. It also acknowledged the breadth of the relevant potential evidence in public health – social, environmental, as well as biological. It pointed to opening the way to a much wider discipline base than had been used hitherto. There were two main elements to the strategy:

> Maximising the use and usefulness of current knowledge to improve public health. This includes selecting current knowledge according to its quality, relevance and potential, synthesising it, making it easily accessible and advocating its use.
>
> Developing and extending the current evidence base to acquire new knowledge to improve public health. This includes identifying the need for research, investing in research and research capacity, and ensuring that the new knowledge which results is integrated into the evidence base and used to its full potential (Department of Health, 2001: 8).

The idea becomes a reality

The then newly established HDA was pinpointed as one of the organisations to be directly involved: 'To this end, the new Health Development Agency (HDA) will have a central role in advising policy-makers on the evidence base for health improvement, and setting standards to guide local policy and practice' (Department of Health, 2001: 15). The HDA was also to be responsible for managing a number of websites to underpin the work, and to liaise with other bodies 'to develop a coordinated approach to the assembly, synthesis and dissemination of public health information' (ibid.: 17). By the autumn of 2001, a programme of work had begun at the HDA, to conduct evidence synthesis and appraisal and to present the findings in an easily digestible form (Mulvihill and Quigley, 2003; Bull, Mulvihill and Quigley, 2003). This programme was undertaken in close collaboration with colleagues in the Department of Health,

EPPI-Centre and CRD. The first project concerned the state of the evidence on accident prevention (Millward, Morgan and Kelly, 2003). Initially the briefings were based on reviews of reviews – finding out what was already known, and synthesising it.

When the first Evidence Briefings were published there was a good deal of scepticism from some academics and practitioners. The idea of reviewing review level evidence was criticised on the grounds that it was too many steps removed from the original primary research to pick up the nuances of the primary studies. Therefore, interpretation would be difficult, and the fidelity of the findings would be in doubt. Some practitioners were also sceptical on the grounds that the kinds of original studies which had been conducted related to issues that were easily measurable and/or were predominantly about downstream individualistic interventions, such as smoking cessation, and therefore did not deal with the wider or social determinants of health, or the fundamental problems of health inequalities.

In fact, the team at the HDA had already produced a policy document for the Department of Health, reviewing the evidence about interventions to reduce health inequalities (Millward, Kelly and Nutbeam, 2003). This had not been a review of reviews. It found that while many papers were published which described the problem of health inequalities, very few actually contained clear policy or practice recommendations about how to deal with the problem. There was a gap between what was known about the problem and what to do about it. As a briefing for the Chief Medical Officer's department in the Department of Health, this policy document was not originally made widely available, but it attracted favourable attention (Petticrew et al., 2004), and was eventually published. It had shown that it was quite possible to conduct powerful evidence reviews of important policy relevance, as well as pointing to a fundamental weakness in the evidence base, including the disconnect between psychologically driven behaviour change approaches to individualistically framed problems and broader foci on the social determinants of health.

However, it was the Evidence Briefings which really broke through the credibility barrier for the HDA. Despite being reviews of reviews, despite being steps removed from the original studies, these syntheses of what was known in a form which was accessible were much appreciated by practitioners and academic colleagues wanting a quick appraisal of the evidence before embarking on new studies, or as an aid to teaching. The Briefings were a ready source of reference. Policy-makers in the Department of Health made much use of them, and they were used in briefings for ministers.

The team at the HDA was not naïve about the limitations of trying to synthesise what was a very limited evidence base, heavily dominated by psychology and epidemiology, firmly facing downstream, and which was in some arenas methodologically very weak. For example, in physical activity, problems of measurement abounded (Hillsdon et al., 2004). Above all, it was clear that the evidence did not speak for itself. It required interpretation by those who knew the evidence and/or practice. The solution which was devised was to establish an advisory group for each topic area which would review the evidence that had been synthesised and summarised by staffers at the HDA, to help in the sense-making process. An overarching topic and methods group was also established to assist in selecting topics to be reviewed and to engage in the interpretation of the material, chaired by one of the Deputy Chief Medical Officers.

The question of economics was also considered by the HDA team. A group of health economists was convened to consider the question of whether the cost utility principles which NICE were using in clinical medicine could be applied to public health. The conclusion was that they could not and that cost conse-quence analysis was a more useful tool for public health (Kelly et al., 2005). This pamphlet attracted a lot of attention. Colleagues from NICE, including several eminent health economists, made it clear – in the spirit of collegial debate – that they disapproved of the argument, and that the QALY and cost–utility analysis remained the gold standard. This gentle academic exchange of ideas was to take a serious turn by the time the next NHS reorganisation was planned and NICE and the HDA were to amalgamate.

However, other events pre-empted that reorganisation, when the Minister with responsibility for public health at the time, Lord Warner, decided that NICE should develop a guideline covering the clinical *and* public health aspects of obesity. The steer from the Minister was that NICE and the HDA should work together on the guideline. The organisations had not collaborated before, and the methods that each was using, while having some things in common, were different. A series of meetings took place between the Guidelines Development Team in NICE and the team in the HDA which had been assigned to work on the obesity project. It was amicably agreed that the methods to be used on the new obesity guideline would be the NICE clinical guideline methods, with NICE addressing clinical aspects, while the HDA team would focus on the pub-lic health and inequalities evidence. This turned out to be an important prov-ing ground, because it showed that the two organisations could work together successfully and a consilience on methods, including health economics, was possible.

NICE and the HDA amalgamate

The obesity guideline was underway when the next NHS reorganisation was announced during 2004. It became clear that that HDA was to be part of a 'bon-fire of the quangos'. Under this cloud, the main work programmes on producing the Evidence Briefings and other publications continued, as did the joint work with NICE on obesity. There was a prolonged period of uncertainty, with posts in the HDA put at risk. It was generally assumed that parts of the HDA would be amalgamated with the Health Protection Agency. In the event that is not what happened. The decision, which few had anticipated, was that NICE would amalgamate with the HDA and would assume responsibility for producing public health guidelines to all intents and purposes, the same as clinical guidelines. Interestingly, precisely this idea – public health evidence-based guidelines – had originally been suggested back in 2001 in the Department of Health Research and Development Strategy (Department of Health, 2001: 15).

On reflection this was a masterstroke. The two organisations were already working together, the methods of review and syntheses could be nuanced, there was potential consilience between the methods, the experience that the HDA had in respect of extending the principles of EBM to public health could be aligned with NICE guideline development methods, and the expertise which the HDA possessed on health inequalities could be applied. And all of this could be brought to bear on producing public health guidelines for the NHS (which still at that time had the main responsibility for public health in England), as well as local authorities and other organisations whose remits extended to disease prevention and health protection.

Almost immediately a list of topics for the NICE public health centre to work on was agreed with the Department of Health. It was decided by the senior team at NICE that to maximise speed and impact, the first two guidelines would be in areas where the HDA had already synthesised the evidence – smoking cessation and the promotion of physical activity. These were followed by the prevention of sexually transmitted infections (including HIV), preventing teenage pregnancy and drug misuse, workplace health promotion, and behaviour change. This list was very disease-oriented and the briefs for the work from the Department of Health had a strongly individualistic and behaviour change orientation. The reconciliation of the tension between the individual and the population approaches became a defining trope for the work which NICE public health did, and especially as it sought to orient the guidance towards tackling health inequalities.

Public health economics

In the meantime, thought had to be given to public health economics. As noted above, the HDA had already published a pamphlet calling into question the idea of the application of cost utility analysis to public health. To consider the issue a number of meetings took place, perhaps the most important of which was when Professor Tony Culyer, eminent health economist and deputy chair at NICE, visited the new public health team at NICE. His argument was that, while the case made in the HDA pamphlet about public health and preventive medicine and QALYs was right, it would not be helpful in making the case for public health. He argued that the QALY would allow for the direct comparison of clinical interventions, such as new pharmaceuticals, with public health interventions like smoking cessation or promoting physical activity. And, very importantly, these would be powerful forces in making the political, economic and policy case for public health. The logic of his argument was compelling and it was therefore agreed that as far as possible the cost utility analysis and QALY values would be calculated for public health topics. These principles were incorporated into the first and subsequent methods manual for public health at NICE (NICE, 2012).

Undertaking economic analysis was challenging as there was limited data concerning costs for any public health interventions or programmes, and so conducting health economic analysis of any kind was initially very insecure. This meant that the evidence base had to be searched far and wide, and in the absence of hard data, the economic analysis had to be based on modelling. This is a well-established economic technique, but it brings further problems, perhaps the most acute of which is the way to incorporate theories of behaviour and behaviour change – always central to this kind of economic modelling – into the equation.

The wisdom of Culyer's words became clear as soon as the first new guidelines were in development. The Centre for Public Health Excellence at NICE had established, as part of its methods procedures, a Public Health Interventions Advisory Committee (PHIAC). At its first meeting, when the evidence on smoking cessation and physical activity were considered, the effectiveness evidence was unequivocal. But the health economics evidence was nothing short of astounding. At that time the threshold which NICE used to assess cost-effectiveness was circa £20,000 per QALY. When the economists presented their calculations about the QALY values on smoking cessation and the promotion of physical activity, they were in the mid-hundreds, quanta below the NICE threshold. In other words, they were highly cost-effective! As the years went by and other guidelines were developed, the vast majority never exceeded the £20,000 threshold and it became possible to mount very good cases for the value for money of public health interventions (Owen and Fischer, 2019).

Whether this has ever really influenced policy makers is doubtful, because recent decades have seen the budgets for public health across England reduced by successive policies of austerity, as well as the diversion of resources into pharmaceuticals and treatments, rather than prevention. But the hard facts of the economics remain. Compared to expenditure on treatments, prevention is very good value for money. This is not of course to argue that treatment budgets should be cut, but rather that prevention should not be overlooked as resources are allocated nationally. The difficulties of applying the QALY to some aspects of public health remain, and the value of using cost consequence analysis for some purposes is not unimportant, but the comparative cost-effectiveness of public health and the demonstration of this is one of NICE's most important contributions.

Health inequalities

One of the projects that had just begun in the HDA when it was amalgamated with NICE was to lead the Evidence and Knowledge Network of the Commission on the Social Determinants of Health for the World Health Organization

(WHO). This work continued in NICE. A staff group from within the public health team at NICE led a global consortium in considering the methodological issues attaching to summarising, synthesising and presenting the global evidence on the social determinants of health. This was to be based on social scientific as well as biomedical evidence. The project was to inform and underpin the other evidence networks globally which were producing the material for the Commission. Between 2005 and 2008 there were various publications (Kelly et al., 2006; 2007) ahead of the final publication of the report by WHO in 2008 (WHO, 2008) exploring the methodological problems. The lessons arising also, very importantly, fed into the public health guidelines development processes in NICE which were underway at the same time (Kelly et al., 2009).

This work for WHO showed that there was a major divide in the evidence base. There was a large amount of evidence showing that the wider determinants of health, like the economy, employment patterns, housing, environmental conditions, poverty, gender relations, and racism, had profound effects on patterns of population health. In short, disadvantage, however it is measured, is strongly associated with poor health. Advantaged circumstances, in contrast, are associated at population level with good health. It does not matter how advantage and disadvantage are operationalised and measured – class, occupation, education, earnings, housing, or place of residence, and it does not matter how health is measured – mortality, morbidity, subjective health state – the results are always the same. There is a health gradient across the population. However, the evidence is primarily associational or correlational and the mechanisms linking the factors together are not much covered, or were not at that time, in the evidence base. This was not to deny the associations are real, but it was to leave open the question of the best way to intervene on the mechanisms, if the causal mechanisms are themselves unclear.

The evidence also showed that the factors which determine health are not necessarily the same as those which drive health inequalities. It is important to distinguish between the different phenomena. Although linked, they are different, and it is vitally important to understand the relationships and the mechanisms operating between the phenomena, and from a policy perspective to recognise that action is needed on both types. This is important in helping to prioritise different policy options (Graham and Kelly, 2004).

It is also clear that different sections of the population respond differently to the same types of interventions. There is differential effectiveness of interventions, which reflect social variation in the population. Two important problems arise as a consequence. Do we have good evidence about differential effectiveness? Do we know enough about the social differences in the population to accurately describe the social variegation in it? The answer to both was, and is, no. While some studies gather data about occupation, age, gender, ethnicity etc. they do not use the data to test for differential effectiveness. Such data are used, in so far as they are collected at all, to test for confounding or to describe baseline characteristics of populations or samples. Further the categories which are used to collect such data are relatively crude and do not collect information in sufficient granularity to describe the rich variegation in populations and the intersectional interactions between the different dimensions of social difference.

It should also be noted that the wider determinants literature is quite disconnected from most of the literature concerning interventions operating at the individual level, principally those studies concerned with behaviour change designed to help people stop smoking, take more exercise, drink less alcohol and consume a healthier diet. These interventions operate within a highly individualistic frame of reference, and seldom address the question of the social determinants, or of health inequities more generally. Of course, across the global evidence base, there are exceptions (Kelly et al., 2023), but in general terms, the separation is profound. It also became apparent in this methodological work for WHO, that the social determinants literature and the behaviour change evidence are *both* disconnected from the world of policy. Both describe the problems extremely well, but neither really address how that evidence can be easily and effectively translated into political action – the 'how to' question remains largely unanswered.

This helped to frame the evidence for the WHO Commission's Report but also in NICE's public health guideline work, as the UK data was a microcosm of the global data with exactly the same fault lines. It also assisted enormously in the deliberations of PHIAC and of the other public health advisory committees.

Interventions and programmes

The public health topics which the Department of Health directed NICE to work on had a heavily individualistic, behaviour change focus. They were also strongly oriented to 'interventions'. The assumption was that a public health activity could be framed as a single, or a series of discrete actions, which might be treated similarly to a pharmaceutical intervention. Of course, there are some matters, like the provision of nicotine replacement therapy, or brief advice about alcohol misuse, which fit this mould. In these areas there were studies, including RCTs, measuring the effect sizes of such interventions, and NICE made use of these. But much of what is in the public health armoury does not consist of single discrete interventions. Instead, they are programmes of activities, or policies designed to facilitate action, usually involving multi-components operating simultaneously – sometimes at the individual level, sometimes at the population level and sometimes both. It is all much fuzzier than the language of discrete interventions implies.

Although there was a constant dialogue between NICE and the Department of Health, as well as with stakeholders, there was a continuous tension between the need to cover broader programmes and the need to specify particular interventions. Initially there was a dual track of work packages in the public health activities in NICE, with a distinction drawn between work which came under the aegis of PHIAC and what were called interventions, and another dealing with broader material. The original guidance on behaviour change was the first to be published from the broader work package (NICE, 2007). The two work streams were eventually merged. It was difficult to maintain the boundaries between the two as there was much overlap, and stakeholders and policy makers did not fully understand the dual track approach. However, difficulties of the intrinsic breadth of public health activity and putting it in a framework which had originated as a way of determining the cost-effectiveness of new pharmaceuticals and treatment guidelines, remained.

The problems with the extant evidence

There were other difficulties. In many arenas there was a dearth of good outcome studies. There were studies which described process, there were descriptions of activities, but answering the questions 'What works, for whom and under what circumstances?' (Pawson and Tilley, 1997) was difficult on the basis of the existing evidence. Further, the evidence, such as it was, was often too imprecise to determine the mechanistic or causal relationship between the intervention *or* programme and the outcomes.

Another problem was the generally poor quality of the studies themselves. The methodological quality of the evidence left much to be desired. No study is ever perfect, but once an appraisal of evidence quality is undertaken, it becomes very clear that even studies that are published in high quality/impact journals, are not always that good. Neither was the pedigree of the group of researchers undertaking the work, or the prestige or ranking of the university where the studies were done, a guide to quality. The task became one of appraising quality *de novo*. The issue is one of deciding the point at which the methodological flaws are so significant as to override the results and lead them to be discarded (Ogilvie et al., 2005). The poor quality of studies was not of course unique to the public health portfolio, and many involved in EBM had given the problem of the quality of studies and making sensible recommendations on the basis of poor evidence considerable attention (Guyatt et al., 2008a; 2008b).

The workable solution which had been devised in EBM was the so-called hierarchy of evidence. The hierarchy divides evidence into that which consisted of meta-analyses, and synthesis of good quality randomised controlled trials as the highest quality of evidence, down to expert opinion as the lowest quality evidence. This was a useful way of considering and appraising a particular type of evidence, and much work has been done to refine definitions and methods to synthesise, evaluate and determine what counts as quality across the hierarchy (Greenhalgh, 2001). The problem that NICE, and before it the HDA team, had faced, was that this is really a hierarchy of methods, not of evidence, and a limited range of methods at that. Outside of the domain of clinical trials, it becomes problematic to use the hierarchy as the *only* guide to assessing the quality of studies. Where possible, the public health team and the review centres around the country which undertook the evidence reviews to support the various guidelines, would use the hierarchy, but in areas where qualitative evidence and studies of social and organisational processes were involved, it was necessary to work to other types of quality appraisal. As time went on, this became easier, as the scientific community and, especially, the social scientific community refined quality appraisal of different types of non-trial-based evidence (Noyes et al., 2022).

What was also very important was that the quality appraisal of the evidence did not drive the strength of recommendations. In short, it was sometimes the case that there was high quality evidence, along whichever of the quality metrics were being used, but this was not necessarily the evidence which answered the most important questions. Sometimes there was poor quality evidence about an important problem. Sometimes there was no evidence at all! This means that judgements about interpreting and applying the evidence, are a good deal more complex than just assessing methodological quality (Kelly and Moore, 2012; Rawlins, 2008).

This gives rise to two questions. The first is about the quality of the evidence itself. How confident can we be that the relationship between the dependent and the independent variable, or between the intervention and/or the programme and the outcomes, are real and free from bias? This is the internal validity question. Of course, this question is premised on an idea that the relationship between the two is real. But we often have very little evidence about mechanisms or precise causal pathways. Further, variables, or interventions or programmes and their outcomes, exist within a complex web of relationships empirically. The notion of one variable acting on another is premised on a particular view of cause, which is derived from pre-Einsteinian physics, not the behavioural and social sciences.

The second question is the external validity question; or more precisely, the transferability question. There may be good evidence derived from a single or a few studies. It shows that a given action has produced highly favourable outcomes where the research was originally conducted. But if we transfer the activity to somewhere else, where there are no researchers undertaking a specific study, and where the context is quite different, will it still work? In one discussion in a guideline development committee the phrase 'Will it work, on a wet Wednesday in Wigan' was suggested, not just for its alliterative qualities, but as a way to get the committee really thinking about the practicalities of real-world implementation and practice.

The judgement process involved is vexing. It is not just that it is a judgement, and individual committee members have to make subjective appraisals, but also that there are no protocols to guide the process. This is in marked contrast to the processes for assessing and appraising empirical data. There are well defined protocols for methods of scientific interpretation, with statistical tests, p values, confidence intervals, and very clear guidance on the way to assess a trial; while allocation to trial arms, blinding of participants, and intention to treat analysis, amongst others, provide markers whereby the quality of the research can be assessed. This helps to guide the process. However, the methods for understanding processes of inference and judgement are less well understood or articulated.

The public health team at NICE resolved the problem by trying to articulate what *a priori* information was being brought to the table by committee members making judgements – was it derived from clinical or practice experience, was it based on other knowledge of research studies, was it based on theoretical or ideological assumptions? This demands expert chairing, and a requirement for persons making the judgements to reflect carefully on their own subjective viewpoints. In several of the published guidelines, it was made quite explicit that there were judgements based on empirical evidence and there were other kinds of judgements which were in play (NICE, 2010a). The aspiration was to be as transparent as possible, something that became all the more imperative when NICE took the decision to hold some of its committee meetings in public, including some of the public health meetings.

The overall idea behind the idea of making judgments explicit was to move away from a formulaic and naively positivistic way of doing EBM. Several scientific papers were published which explored the issues and the philosophical background. The tensions between Humean rationalism and empiricism (Hume, 1748/2007), and Kantian analytic and synthetic thinking (Kant, 1781/2007), are old epistemological problems, and it was very interesting to note how these problems remained front and centre in EBM (Kelly and Moore, 2012). The idea that evidence does not speak for itself – it always requires interpretation – is absolutely right, and while simple to say proves to be hard to put into practice.

The problem of values

Once the decision had been taken to do health economics using cost utility analysis, a predictable disjunction emerged in relation to producing cost-effective guidelines which at the same time addressed health inequalities. Cost utility analysis is, as is all economic utility analysis, rooted in utilitarian thinking. There will always be losers in utilitarian market systems, but the idea is that overall, society at large benefits. The principle of cost-effectiveness runs into a problem, namely cost-effective for whom? When Alan Williams was developing the principles of cost utility analysis and its application to health, the main goal was to come up with a fair and efficient society wide resource allocation model. The solution was the QALY, derived from cost utility principles, which provides a metric which allows for the comparison of value for money for the payer – the exchequer in the UK. It is possible to compare pharmaceutical interventions with a surgical intervention, or with any kind of intervention. Inequalities in health, and certainly solutions to ameliorate them, may not fit easily into the QALY logic.

For example, an intervention to provide smoking cessation services, may on average be cost-effective, but once the intervention has to be nuanced and targeted to reach communities where need is greatest, but which are resistant to services, or where there is distrust of efforts by authorities of various kinds to change things, the actual delivery costs in time, effort and money become greater. The idea that the resource allocation problem is solved is called into question.

The issue was resolved in the public health work stream by focussing on overall average population QALY values, rather than specific population groups, in the full knowledge that in fine-grained detail, not all interventions were cost-effective – either to the same degree, or at all – once applied to certain population groups. This was made the easier because the level of detail about differential effectiveness in sub-groups in the population was itself so limited, that it would have been extremely difficult to do the calculations with sufficient granularity to make accurate calculations anyway. It was this kind of reasoning that had led the original HDA pamphlet on the economics of public health to question the usefulness of the QALY in that arena (Kelly et al., 2005). It is probably also the case that when the NICE public health guidelines appeared, even the most controversial ones, it was never the health economics that attracted attention from critics, even though there was a significant degree of uncertainty about the underlying principles. An uneasy truce between cost utility utilitarian thinking and egalitarian principles prevailed.

The media and political responses

Much of what NICE did in public health had considerable political and media profile. Guidelines derived from the evidence, even the limited evidence NICE had initially at its disposal, often ran against the grain of prevailing governmental orthodoxies. So NICE found itself facing a new set of controversies. This was not new for the organisation, having already had to deal with the push-back against its sometimes-controversial recommendations about funding new drugs. With public health, NICE now found itself at odds not just with the pharmaceutical industry, but also with the advertising, food, and alcohol industries, the right-wing media and think tanks, academic sceptics and government itself.

The first skirmish was however, pretty low profile. In the second piece of guidance produced, on the promotion of physical activity, one of its recommendations ran counter to one of the policy streams favoured at that time by ministers. Pedometers were all the rage, and there was a widely held view that they would help people do more exercise and walk further. The (limited) evidence did not support the idea that pedometers were an evidence-based cost-effective long-term intervention. Officials were despatched to NICE to see if some kind of compromise could be arranged. But NICE held its ground, and the government advice on pedometers was quietly shelved. The evidence-base on wearable devices of all kinds has increased considerably since 2006, and NICE's recommendations are now different. But this showed that even something as apparently innocuous as a pedometer could be a source of considerable political discomfort.

The public health programme continued to produce a string of guidelines over the next four years, and although there was sometimes hostile commentary in the media, and accusations of nanny-statism levelled at NICE, the outputs became increasingly well known. However, the relative calm was shattered in 2010. NICE had been working on a guideline on the prevention of alcohol use disorders and harmful drinking, and publication was due in early to mid 2010 (NICE, 2010a). There were recommendations in the guideline about brief interventions, there was material on preventing harm, and controlling availability. However, there was also a section relating to minimum unit pricing. A general election was called for that year, in May, and under the arrangement called in the Civil Service 'purdah', NICE would not publish anything, nor make any public statements in the weeks leading up to the election. The guideline was, however, ready before the election was called.

Careful thought was given to the timing of its release. It could have been published before the election and before 'purdah', but in consultation with Department of Health officials, it was agreed that a release after the election would optimise the profile of the guidance. It was suggested by civil servants that there would likely be new ministers in office, even if the governing party did not change, and they would be looking for fresh ideas. This would, it was suggested, be ideal for making the new alcohol guidance public.

However, on the day of release and immediately afterwards, the response of the ministers in the new Coalition Government was immediate and very hostile. The new Secretary of State for Health had made very clear, even before the election, that he was opposed to minimum unit pricing. He was as good as his word, and the day following the release of the guideline, the Department of Health issued a briefing, rejecting the conclusions that the Guideline Development Committee in NICE had reached. The alcohol industry also weighed in with its arguments and the guideline had, as a consequence, an enormous amount of coverage in the media – broadcast and print (see e.g. Laurance, 2010).

Around the same time a guideline on the prevention of coronary heart disease was also published (NICE, 2010b). This emphasised specific examples of upstream factors – wider or social determinants of health – and heart health, and impacts on health inequalities. It covered topics like the Common Agricultural Policy, marketing, food production, and many upstream levers to bring about health improvement. New ministers saw it as an encroachment on the elected government's prerogative to make policy. The guideline did not of course make policy, it simply pointed to a framework of upstream evidence-based actions that could have population benefits, especially in relation to health inequalities.

NICE did not retract either the alcohol or the heart disease guideline, and at the time of preparing this chapter, they are still current on the NICE website. But there were considerable ramifications. The new Secretary of State indicated, a few weeks later, that the NICE public health programme was to be curtailed and the consequence was that NICE should not in future deal with, or make policy recommendations: in effect meaning anything concerning the wider determinants of health and health inequalities. A number of programmes of work were cut, and the briefs coming from the Department of Health were thereafter considerably more anodyne. It takes a degree of courage to stand firm against such political pressure. But the Chief Executive and the Chair at NICE (Andrew Dillon and Mike Rawlins) stood behind the guidelines, as they had done in the case of previous controversial decisions about pharmaceuticals. The corporate view in NICE was that if the proper protocols for searching the evidence base, appraising the evidence, and making recommendations had been followed, it was absolutely right to defend the recommendations of its properly constituted independent advisory committees.

Interestingly the evidence relating to minimum unit pricing of alcohol is now stronger than it was in 2010, and the Common Agricultural Policy disappeared as a result of Brexit. Upstream policies to effect change and improvements in public health are if anything, even more imperative than they were a decade or more ago – we have seen a stalling of the long-run improvements in life expectancy, and since 2010 heath inequalities have widened. The reluctance of government to embrace a population approach to health improvement including on these two topics, remains part at least, of the explanation for this.

Of course, public health is and always has been political. Arguments in favour of personal liberty as against restriction in the interests of protecting health, are as old as efforts in early modern Europe (and probably earlier) to control the spread of plague (McNeill, 1977). They echo down the years in efforts to protect the population from infections like cholera and typhoid and to build sewers and provide clean water, through to efforts to improve housing conditions and child nutrition in the twentieth century (Jackson, 2014). Efforts to restrict the sales of tobacco which (albeit with considerable time lag) followed in the wake of the discovery of the link between exposure to cigarette smoke and lung cancer and other serious disease, were always political. The conflict which followed NICE's publication of its guidance on alcohol is simply a recent manifestation of the recurring liberty versus restriction debate, a debate which became pronounced once again during the Covid-19 pandemic.

The solution may seem hard to find, but one way of thinking about the issue is to acknowledge the two realms of evidence and politics. They are different. The role of the scientist is to do the utmost to provide the best available evidence and its interpretation, but also to acknowledge its limits. The political role is not just to make decisions, but to make decisions which the electorate will find palatable, and of course to help bolster subsequent political electoral support. In the case of the alcohol guideline, a more measured response from government might have been to thank NICE for the evidence-based guideline, but to argue that at that particular time, it did not fit with government policy, nor was it likely to be acceptable to the general public. This would not have led to a showdown with the scientists and a feeble effort to argue that they were wrong. The fact of course is that the evidence is the evidence, and although ministers may not like it, it stands the test of time in a way that ministers do not.

That said, the *modus operandi* for public health after the dust had settled was considerably lower-key. The development of public health guidelines was, after 2014, absorbed into a general guideline development programme in NICE, and there have been few occasions since when NICE public health work excited the ire of ministers. However, what was lost was an independent and respected voice that was evidence-based and which sought to place health inequalities front and centre. The move away from focusing on the social determinants of health within NICE may prove to have been a significant mistake. When the COVID 19 pandemic enveloped the world, and as jurisdictions world-wide struggled to find practical and policy solutions, the value of an independent evidence-based machine to rapidly review and develop guidelines was sorely missed in the UK. Of course, as everywhere, the UK had a plethora of experts, some of whom were in the various advisory committees advising government. In reality, there were many competing voices, inside and outside of official committees, mostly seeking to advance particular interpretations of the science – precisely the situation so trenchantly criticised by Archie Cochrane decades before. A body separate from the machinery of government, unshackled from the politics of the pandemic, was missing – a role NICE public health could have played.

Conclusion

The problem of inequalities in health has not gone away. The evidence base about interventions is certainly better than it was in 2001 when HDA began its work, and some of the deficits in the evidence mentioned above, have to some extent been remedied. However, in spite of evidential improvements, there remains a gap, which is about how to get this evidence into the hands of those who need it, and in a way that they are able to use at local level (Atkins et al., 2017). So, while the evidence now is good at identifying what needs to be done, how to do it remains to be demonstrated. This of course was something which NICE in its clinical guidelines programme had long been aware of, but it was thrown into stark relief by the public health work stream at NICE. It is now clear that above and beyond the evidence on effectiveness and cost-effectiveness, there is another type of evidence, that researchers seldom write about, which is the 'how to'. This exists, but in the grey literature, in the literature of the management sciences, and in historical accounts of past successes and failures. As we move forward, perhaps one task for NICE for its next 25 years, is to develop ways of corralling such evidence and synthesising it in a way that will be of use and value to the front-line practitioners whose daily job is about making it happen.

References

Atkins, L., Kelly, M.P., Littleford, C., Leng, G. and Michie, S. (2017) 'Reversing the pipeline? Implementing public health evidence-based guidance in English local government', *Implementation Science*, 12(63).

Bull, J., Mulvihill, C. and Quigley, R. (2003) *Prevention of Low Birth Weight: Assessing Effectiveness of Smoking Cessation and Nutritional Intervention. Evidence Briefing.* London: Health Development Agency.

Chalmers, I., Dickersin, K. and Chalmers, T.C. (1992) 'Getting to grips with Archie Cochrane's agenda: All randomised controlled trials should be registered and reported', *British Medical Journal* 305(6857), pp.786–87.

Cochrane, A.L. (1972) *Effectiveness and Efficiency: Random Reflections on Health Services.* London: British Medical Journal/Nuffield Provincial Hospitals Trust.

Department of Health (2001) *A Research and Development Strategy for Public Health.* London: Department of Health.

Egger, M., Higgins, J.P.T. and Davey Smith, G. (2022) *Systematic Reviews in Health Research: Meta-Analysis in Context.* 3rd edn, London: BMJ Books.

Graham, H. and Kelly, M.P. (2004) *Health Inequalities: Concepts, Frameworks and Policy.* London: Health Development Agency.

Greenhalgh, T. (2001) *How to Read a Paper: The Basics of Evidence-Based Medicine.* London: BMJ Books.

Guyatt, G., Oxman, A.D., Vist, G.E., Kunz, R., Falck-Ytter, Y., Alonso-Coello, P. and Schunemann, H.J., for the GRADE Working Group. (2008a) 'GRADE: an emerging consensus on rating quality of evidence and strength of recommendations', *British Medical Journal*, 336, pp.924–26.

Guyatt, G., Oxman, A.D., Kunz, R., Falck-Ytter, Y., Vist, G.E., Liberati, A., Schunemann, H.J. and the GRADE Working Group (2008b) 'Going from evidence to recommendations', *British Medical Journal* 336, pp.1049–51.

Hillsdon, M., Foster, C., Naidoo, B. and Crombie, H. (2004) *The Effectiveness of Public Health Interventions for Increasing Physical Activity among Adults: A Review of Reviews.* London: Health Development Agency.

Hume, D. (1748) *An Enquiry Concerning Human Understanding*, edited with an introduction by Millican, P. (2007) Oxford: Oxford University Press.

Jackson, L. (2014) *Dirty Old London: The Victorian Fight Against Filth.* New Haven: Yale University Press.

Kant, I. (1781) *The Critique of Pure Reason*, translated by Kemp Smith, N., with an introduction by Caygill, H. (2007) Basingstoke: Palgrave Macmillan.

Kelly, M.P. (2018) The need for a rationalist turn in Evidence-Based Medicine, *Journal of Evaluation in Clinical Practice*, 24, pp.1158–65.

Kelly, M.P., and Moore, T.A. (2012) 'The judgement process in Evidence-Based Medicine and Health Technology Assessment', *Social Theory and Health*, 10(1), pp.1–19.

Kelly, M.P., McDaid, D., Ludbrook, A. and Powell, J. (2005) *Economic Appraisal of Public Health Interventions.* London: Health Development Agency.

Kelly, M.P., Bonnefoy, J., Morgan, A. and Florenzano, F. (2006) *The Development of the Evidence Base about the Social Determinants of Health.* Geneva: WHO Commission on the Social Determinants of Health.

Kelly, M.P., Morgan, A., Bonnefoy, J., Butt, J. and Bergman, V. (2007) *The Social Determinants of Health: Developing an Evidence Base for Political Action. Final Report to the World Health Organization Commission on the Social Determinants of Health.* Available at: https://cdn.who.int/media/docs/default-source/documents/social-determinants-of-health/measurement-and-evidence-knowledge-network-final-report-2007.pdf (Accessed 22 March 2023).

Kelly, M.P., Stewart, E., Morgan, A., Killoran, A., Fischer, A., Threlfall, A. and Bonnefoy, J. (2009) 'A conceptual framework for public health: NICE's emerging approach', Public Health 123(1), pp.e14–e20.

Kelly, M.P., Arora, A., Banerjee, A., Birch, J.M., Ekeke, N., Kuhn, I., Brayne, C., Ford, J., Aquino, M.R.J. and Capper, B. (2023) *Review of the Contribution of Behavioural Science to Addressing the Social and Wider Determinants of Health: Evidence Review.* Geneva: World Health Organization.

Laurance, J. (2010) 'Government rejects health watchdog's alcohol policy', *The Independent* (2 June). Available at: https://www.independent.co.uk/life-style/health-and-families/health-news/government-rejects-health-watchdog-s-alcohol-policy-by-health-watchdog-1988869.html (Accessed 7 February 2023).

McNeill, W.H. (1977) *Plagues and Peoples.* New York: Doubleday.

Millward, L.M., Kelly, M.P. and Nutbeam, D. (2003) *Public Health Interventions Research: The Evidence.* London: Health Development Agency.

Millward, L.M., Morgan, A. and Kelly, M.P. (2003) *Prevention and Reduction of Accidental Injury in Children and Older People.* Evidence Briefing. London: Health Development Agency.

Mulvihill, C. and Quigley, R. (2003) *The Management of Obesity and Overweight: An Analysis of Reviews of Diet, Physical Activity and Behavioural Approaches.* Evidence briefing. London: Health Development Agency.

NHS Centre for Reviews and Dissemination, University of York (1995) *Review of the Research on the Effectiveness of Health Services Interventions to Reduce Variations in Health,* CRD Report 3.

NICE (2007) 'Behaviour change at population, community and individual levels'. Public Health Guidance 6. London: NICE.

NICE (2010a) 'Alcohol use disorders: preventing harmful drinking'. Public Health Guidance 24. London: NICE.

NICE (2010b) 'Prevention of cardiovascular disease at population level'. Public Health Guidance 25. London: NICE.

NICE (2012) 'Methods for the development of NICE public health guidance'. PMG4. 3rd edn., London: NICE.

Noyes, J., Booth, A., Cargo, M., Flemming, K., Harden, A., Harris, J., Garside, R., Hannes, K., Pantoja, T. and Thomas, J. (2022) 'Qualitative evidence', in Higgins J.P.T., Thomas J., Chandler J., Cumpston M., Li T., Page M.J. and Welch V.A. (eds). *Cochrane Handbook for Systematic Reviews of Interventions,* ver. 6.3. Available at www.training.cochrane.org/handbook (Accessed 26 March 2023).

Ogilvie, D., Egan, M., Hamilton, V. and Petticrew, M. (2005) 'Systematic reviews of health effects of social interventions: 2: best available evidence: how low should you go?', *Journal of Epidemiology and Community Health,* 59(10), pp.886–92.

Owen, L. and Fischer, A. (2019) 'The cost-effectiveness of public health interventions examined by the National Institute for Health and Care Excellence from 2005 to 2018', *Public Health;* 169(Apr), pp.151–62.

Pawson, R. and Tilley, N. (1997) *Realistic Evaluation.* London: Sage.

Petticrew, M., Whitehead, M., Macintyre, S.J., Graham, H. and Egan, M. (2004) 'Evidence for public health policy on inequalities: 1: the reality according to policy makers', *Journal of Epidemiology and Community Health,* 58(10), pp.811–16.

Rawlins, M. (2008) *De Testimonio: On the Evidence for Decisions About the Use of Therapeutic Interventions.* The Harvean Oration of 2008. London: Royal College of Physicians.

Sackett, D.L., Rosenberg, W.M.C., Gray J.A.M., Haynes R.B. and Richardson, W.S. (1996) 'Evidence-based medicine: What it is and what it is not', *British Medical Journal,* 312(7023), pp.71–72.

Swann, C., Falce, C., Morgan, A., Kelly, M.P., Powell, G., Carmona, C., Taylor, L. and Taske N. (2005) *HDA Evidence Base: Process and Quality Standards Manual for Evidence Briefings.* 3rd edn. London: Health Development Agency.

The Evidence-Based Medicine Working Group (1992) 'Evidence-Based Medicine. A New Approach to Teaching the Practice of Medicine', *Journal of the American Medical Association,* 268(17), pp.2420–25.

WHO (2008) *Closing the Gap in a Generation: Health Equity Through Action on the Social Determinants of Health.* Geneva: WHO.

Zaza, S., Briss, P.A., and Harris, K.W. (eds) (2005) *The Guide to Community Preventive Services: What Works to Promote Health?* New York: Oxford University Press.

8 Public involvement at NICE

Evolution, not revolution

*Sophie Staniszewska and
Sophie Söderholm Werkö*

Introduction

In this chapter we review 25 years of patient and public involvement and engagement at NICE. NICE has involved patients, service users, carers and the public, including voluntary, charitable and community organisations, since its inception. We track key developments and highlight important milestones.

While the terms 'patient and public involvement' and 'public involvement' have been used by NICE, NICE is now starting to use 'public involvement and engagement'. We will use the term patient and public involvement and engagement to reflect national and international perspectives. In some contexts, we use public involvement for brevity.

Our reflections are based on a review of relevant NICE documents, peer-reviewed papers, the perspectives of NICE colleagues, our direct experience of working with NICE as external collaborators, and our expertise in the field of patient and public involvement, drawing on the underpinning evidence base. We did not have access to internal NICE documents. We have reflected on our perspective in writing this chapter. We are external to NICE but have worked closely with different teams in NICE. Our perspective is influenced by our expertise and experience. Sophie Staniszewska is an academic with a focus on building the evidence base of patient and public involvement and engagement and Sophie Söderholm Werkö is an academic and HTA agency representative, having been responsible for the PPI activities at the agency. It is an account of the evolution of patient and public involvement over 25 years with our external eye.

We consider public involvement at NICE through our academic and agency lens, considering areas where less progress has been made and where NICE could develop public involvement in the future. For example, NICE predominantly views involvement and engagement as a 'doing' activity, rather than an activity that can also generate evidence through research and publication. We acknowledge that such an evidence-informed approach to public involvement is still developing in the sector, but we would encourage NICE to embrace such an approach to public involvement, reflecting the value NICE places on

DOI: 10.4324/9781003501268-8

evidence-based health and social care. We also recognise the importance of consistent leadership in the development of the Public Involvement Programme (PIP) team. This constancy of people, alongside the team's organisational knowledge, its wider expertise, and its international social capital, have all contributed to strengthening patient and public involvement and engagement across NICE (see Chapter 3).

Two key principles have driven NICE's approach to patient and public involvement (NICE, 2023b):

1. *'That lay people, and organisations representing their interests, have opportunities to contribute to developing NICE guidance, advice and quality standards, and support their implementation, and*
2. *that, because of this contribution, NICE guidance and other products have a greater focus and relevance for the people most directly affected by NICE's recommendations.'*

Our overall perspective is that patient and public involvement and engagement at NICE is a success story and there is much to celebrate. Patients, the public and communities have become an embedded part of NICE activity. More broadly, NICE has influenced many agencies and organisations, nationally and internationally, in how they have developed their own strategic direction in relation to involvement and engagement, and importantly provided legitimacy for those involvement activities.

Before we turn to the beginnings of involvement and engagement at NICE, it is important to consider what we mean by patient and public involvement and engagement.

Introduction to patient and public involvement and engagement

Patient and public involvement and engagement has become an important area of activity within many areas of health and social care practice. In essence it usually refers to some form of partnership with patients, carers and service users of public contributors. A range of terms and definitions exist, but for the purpose of this chapter we will use the term patient and public involvement and engagement (and occasionally public involvement for brevity) to reflect national and international perspectives, recognising NICE now uses public involvement and engagement to reflect its broader remit around social care and public health. We recognise that the focus of patient involvement can differ from public involvement, as patients bring life experience to the fore, and public contributors often take a broader societal view not necessarily based on lived experience (Street et al., 2020). These two groups have the potential to express very different and sometimes opposite views (McCabe and Round, 2019). We also note that patient and public involvement is different from patients who are participants or subjects in research studies, providing their experiences and perspectives on health conditions or health systems. This is also different from the role patients can play as active collaborators or partners, shaping the aims and interpretation of a study or activity that contributes to the evidence NICE ultimately evaluates. The intention behind patient and public involvement and engagement at NICE is one of collaborative partnership, with patients, service users, carers, publics and communities working closely with staff and others on a range of NICE activities.

The evolution of public involvement at NICE: The early years

Patient and public involvement and engagement was a core activity when NICE was established in 1999. The College of Health was commissioned to lead patient involvement as part of the National Clinical Guidelines and Audit Involvement Programme and later moved into NICE in 2003 as employed staff members (personal communication, Victoria Thomas, 2009). The commitment to embedding involvement and engagement was reflected in an early paper by Marcia Kelson, the first Head of the NICE Patient Involvement Unit, who wrote 'the National Institute for Health and Clinical Excellence (NICE) has made a substantial and strategic commitment to engaging patients and patient advocates in preparing its guidance, which includes technology appraisal guidance' (Kelson, 2005). The desire to involve patients partly came from the Bristol Baby Heart scandal (Dyer, 2001)[1] and the determination that patients and carers would always be listened to, and their views and experiences acted on, a relatively unusual position internationally at that time. The Patient Involvement Unit worked to develop not only principles of involvement, developed in part from work undertaken by the College of Health and Medical and Nursing Royal Colleges, but also concrete opportunities for involving patients and the public in the work of NICE (Kelson, 2005).

One of the first activities with patients included was the first technology appraisal 'An overview and guidance on the extraction of wisdom teeth'

1 See https://en.wikipedia.org/wiki/Bristol_heart_scandal

(NICE 2000, appendix c Wisdom Teeth Removal). This was the first time that lay members were included in an appraisal panel, representing a significant milestone that provided a foundation for the patient and public involvement seen in health technology assessment today. In addition to patients, the role of patient organisations was strengthened with the establishment of 'Patients Involved in NICE' (PIN) in 2000 as an independent coalition of individuals from patient organisations, now represented by a successor organisation led from within NICE.

The Patient and Public Involvement Programme (PPIP) was formally established alongside the National Collaborating Centre for Mental Health's first guideline on schizophrenia in 2002, focusing on diagnoses and treatment and including a patient version of the guideline. The guideline included recommendations about good practice, such as the importance of the clinician conveying optimism to the patient when discussing their diagnosis (personal communication, Victoria Thomas, 2009). This represented early acknowledgement of the need to consider the patient perspective. In addition, this work identified the need for patients and public contributors to understand the methods NICE used, to support their active involvement and contribution. This led to the development of formal lay training in guideline methodology which was launched in 2002. Such training is now the cornerstone of many patient and public activities, but was relatively rare in 2002.

NICE Citizens Council

A key development within NICE in 2002 was the establishment of the NICE Citizens Council which aimed to provide NICE with a public perspective on the overarching moral and ethical issues that NICE needed to consider when producing guidance. It was made up of members of the public, broadly representative of the UK population and operated through a citizens' jury style meeting to explore questions set by NICE (NICE, 2013). As Dolan, Tsuchiya and Wailoo stated in 2003, 'NICE recognised that its decisions had two components, technical facts, and values. Technical experts are used to address the former (issues such as the cost-effectiveness of a given technology), whereas citizens are called upon to advise about the latter (the set of social value judgments that are used to show how the cost-effectiveness threshold might vary according to certain patients' characteristics, such as age).' While supportive of the Council, Dolan, Tsuchiya and Wailoo (2003) criticised the types of questions that were put to it, arguing for the need for clear and focused questions to minimise ambiguity. The importance of deliberative dialogue in the work of the Citizens Council was explored by

Davies, Barnett and Wetherell (2006). They considered the practical realities behind the focus on deliberation and challenged policymakers and academics to develop a range of approaches to democratic innovation. The NICE Citizens Council has over time considered questions of relevance to NICE. For example, at its meeting in January 2013, the Citizens Council considered the question: 'What aspects of benefit, cost and need should NICE take into account when developing social care guidance?' The Council considered whether the methodology used for assessing health care intervention costs can be used in social care. The response to this was, 'broadly, "no" – current ways of measuring health and aspects of social care will not suffice. NICE needs to develop new methods and processes for social care because there are more differences than similarities' (NICE, 2013). The potential for the public to contribute to such methodological advances was lost when the Council became dormant for a period and then was abolished. Public input re-emerged as 'NICE Listens,' which is a new programme of public engagement, developed to give NICE an understanding of public opinion on moral, ethical, and social value issues (NICE, 2023a). While welcome, there remains an important need to significantly strengthen patient and public involvement in methodological development (as part of involvement and engagement).

Patient and public involvement and engagement in NICE activities

The early 2000s witnessed many milestones where patients and public contributors were involved with a range of NICE actvities for the first time. We had already seen early public involvement in NICE guideline development, which was reviewed by the World Health Organization in 2006, with some important recommendations. These included a suggestion that NICE should undertake comparative evaluations of how consumers and other stakeholders are involved in NICE activities. In addition, the extent of involving individuals within stakeholder organisations should be assessed and consideration should be given to supporting strategies to improve such involvement (WHO Europe, 2006).

Another landmark was the publication of the first interventional procedures guidance on uterine artery embolisation for fibroids in 2010 (NICE, 2010). The Patient and Public Involvement Programme patient surveys formed part of the evidence base and the Interventional Procedures Comittee included lay members. A patient version of the guidance was also published, enabling access to information by the wider public, a development in enabling the public to understand and implement the evidence in their own context. This is no longer standard practice and represents a backward step.

In 2009 NICE launched the Medical Technologies Evaluation Programme to provide rapid assessment of new and innovative medical devices and diagnostics. NICE medical technologies guidance looked at clinical effectiveness and cost impact (as opposed to conducting a full cost-effectiveness analysis). Involvement included two lay members sitting on the committee, and expert testimony was provided by patient organsations via questionnaires and statements. In 2010, the Diagnostics Assessment Programme was launched to enable diagnostic assessment of multiple technologies in one assessment, including cost-effectiveness analysis, again with two lay members sitting on the committee. This membership was supplemented by a patient specialist committee member who was recruited for each individual topic to bring specific lived experience to each assessment. The first diagnostics guidance was then published in 2011 (NICE, 2011a). Through each of these areas of activity, important patient and public perspectives were provided, gradually strengthening the importance of patient input into the work of NICE (Staniszewska and Werkö, 2017).

Developing patient and public involvement and engagement in public health and social care

The extension of NICE's remit to include other substantive areas such as public health and social care provided opportunities for innovation in the way patient and the public were involved, for example by extending this role to service users and carers. In 2005 the Health Development Agency joined forces with NICE to produce public health guidelines and involved 'community members', rather than patients, reflecting the broader population level audience for public health guidance (see Chapter 7). There were three or more community members for each topic, and fieldwork to develop a broader understanding of how the guidance would be received, typically involving voluntary community groups. This new focus led to a significant change in the culture and approach of NICE as an organisation, as broader community perspectives were sought (personal communication, Victoria Thomas, 2009).

Guidelines

Guidelines are tools for improving the quality of health and social care and have been a mainstay of NICE's work, with the publication of a range of guidance created with patients and the public. The NICE website states that NICE guidance aims to improve quality by providing health and social care professionals, and patients and the public, with the information they need to make decisions about treatment and care. In addition, it outlines the range of ways in which patients, service users, carers and the public can be involved directly in producing or promoting NICE guidance, quality standards and other products as formal members of NICE committees and working groups. They can also be involved in NICE's work by commenting, through their organisations, on draft versions of NICE guidance scopes and draft recommendations, and by submitting evidence.

The active involvement of patients in guidelines started in 2002 (personal communication, Victoria Thomas, 2009). In 2004 NICE commissioned the first consultation to obtain the views and experiences of children and young people for a diabetes guideline. The National Children's Bureau recruited children and young people and ran the consultation workshop. This was followed by the first evaluation of PPI in guidelines in 2005.

The broadening of guidelines into other areas was also seen the same year when NICE took on responsibility for public health guidelines. This change had a significant impact on NICE as an organisation broadening its perspective of what a guideline could include (see Chapter 7). It also widened the sorts of organisations which had a stakeholder interest to areas such as housing, environment and education.

In addition to the national focus, the PIP team members have made important contributions to the international guideline development community through the Guideline International Network Patient and Public Involvement working group (GIN Public). They contributed to a paper that set out priorities for patient and public involvement in guidelines identified by participating agencies during a workshop (Boivin et al., 2010). These included the need for research that focused on synthesising existing knowledge and experience to provide guideline developers with an overview of existing methods for involving patients and the public. The group also identified international collaboration priorities such as developing common international standards and frameworks for patient and public involvement development and evaluation that could be adapted to local contexts. The group concluded that greater international collaboration and research were needed to strengthen existing knowledge and evaluation in guideline development.

In 2012 NICE launched the Patient Experience Guideline, which drew on the Warwick Patient Experience Framework as the evidence base from which practice recommendations were developed (Staniszewska et al., 2014). This guidance was important because it recognised patient experience as a form of patient-based evidence, which should be considered alongside clinical and economic forms of evidence in the development of guidance for high quality patient care (Staniszewska and Werkö, 2017). Unusually the guideline development group also included six patients (rather than two) who were actively involved in shaping the themes, recommendations and quality standards. Alongside the Patient Experience Guideline the mental health guideline was developed with significant user input, including a service user co-chair of the guideline development group (NICE, 2011b: NICE, 2012).

Guidelines in social care

In 2012 the Health and Social Care Act gave NICE a new remit for social care with guidelines produced within a culture of co-production which offered very different ways of working and valued a broader range of evidence. Following the Act, the name of the Patient and Public Involvement Programme changed to the Public Involvement Programme in April 2013. The focus on social care led to innovations such as adapted easy to read versions and tailored support for people with learning disabilities on guideline committees (and workshops for recruiting people to the committees). Another innovation was a young people's reference panel for child abuse and neglect. Social care enabled NICE to broaden the boundaries for involvement and the ways in which this worked. The collaboration with the Social Care Institute for Excellence (SCIE) from 2013 supported a co-production approach to the development of guidelines with a service users chair and significant service user representation. This was particularly evident in the development of the Social Care Experience Guideline (NICE, 2018) which drew on the Patient Experience Guideline published in 2012. In reviewing evidence for the guideline, the research team noted studies that had involved service users, an important approach to understanding the extent to which the evidence that underpins a NICE guideline has involvement and engagement at its heart.

In 2017 guidance on antimicrobial resistance was published with a new approach amounting to a suite of guidance on a shared topic. This new way of working focused on finding patients who could speak about a broad range of topics within a particular clinical area, providing a variety of perspectives, not just specific expertise on a particular condition.

The focus on patient experiences continued with the production of guidance focused on the experiences of babies, children and young people (NICE, 2021a). This guideline aimed to describe what a good patient experience for those under 18 could look like and make recommendations on how this can be achieved. The guideline recognised that parents and carers play a role and, where appropriate, their views were considered as the guideline was developed. However NICE also made provision for hearing from children and young people because it was essential for them to establish their views, values and preferences in relation to experience of care. The guideline development recognised that the views of their parents and guardians were not proxies and indeed may be in contradiction to what the children wanted. All the NICE guidelines focused on patient experience contain the tacit assumption that this is a form of evidence, and highlight the vital role that patients, carers and public contributors play in identifying the thematic areas covered, and in creating the recommendations for good practice.

The Covid pandemic created significant challenges for patient and public involvement and engagement at NICE. The Covid-19 rapid guidelines developed by NICE included voluntary and community organisation contributions, despite short deadlines, but made possible by the high quality relationships the Public Involvement Team had previously developed. The Long Covid joint publication with Scottish Intercollegiate Guidelines Network (SIGN) included patient information about Covid. The challenges of Covid meant that the PIP team had to provide significant support for virtual patient and public involvement through the provision of Zoom training, equipment and support for lay members. The team also provided lay member training online with the development of a first batch of online training modules, followed by the second batch in 2021. This reflexive response to the pandemic enabled continued patient and public input into NICE guidance and demonstrated the potential for online forms of involvement.

Shared decision-making

The importance of collaborative partnerships with patients and the public has also been reflected in the work NICE has undertaken on shared decision-making, based on the *NHS Constitution for England*, which states that 'patients, with their families and carers, where appropriate, will be involved in and consulted on all decisions about their care and treatment'. Building on the track record that NICE has achieved in publishing guidance on experiences, it developed a guideline focused on shared decision-making (NICE, 2021b). Shared decision-making emphasises a collaborative approach, promoting ways for healthcare professionals and people using services to work together to make decisions about treatment and care. The guideline covers how to make shared decision-making part of everyday care settings. It includes recommendations on training, communicating risk, benefits and consequences and how to use decision aids. The focus on shared decision-making had enabled NICE to draw on knowledge developed by the European Patients' Academy (EUPATI) to build patient engagement through education as a core component of the approach. EUPATI was established across Europe in 2012 to provide education and training to patients and their advocates. As Thomas says 'initiatives like EUPATI have broken new ground in terms of patients' education and training opportunities. Taking that back into decision-making bodies such as NICE can lead to a greater focus on the issues that matter most to patients' (personal communication, Victoria Thomas, 2009).

Health technology assessment

NICE's remit, from its establishment in 1999, was to create consistent clinical guidelines, and to end rationing of treatment by postcode by providing guidance on new drugs and technologies for use in NHS in England. The technology appraisals NICE has produced since its very start encompass 25 years of experience in health technology assessment (HTA); with different levels of patient involvement included. One of the core principles in involvement in HTA at NICE has been, and still is, to involve people with lived experience of the treatment under consideration or health condition and their families and carers (NICE, 2020).

An important prerequisite for the inclusion and evolution early on of patient involvement in HTA at NICE was the underpinning principle and commitment to including the expertise, experiences and perspectives of lay people, patients, carers and patient organisations. The Values and Quality Standards for patient involvement in HTA, subsequently developed by the Health Technology Assessment International (HTAi) Patient and Citizen Involvement Interest Group, benefited from the input of NICE's PIP team.

The first type of patient involvement in HTA at NICE was simply to recruit lay members to the HTA committees (this is still the case today). Their role is to take a general view on the topic in question and bring the perspectives of people who use health services to HTA decision-making. They should reflect on the patient evidence that is presented to them and emphasise that evidence in committee discussions. From the beginning, NICE went further than what was considered best practice at the time (e.g. one lay member on a committee in 2001), and decided that there should be a minimum of two lay members on each committee at NICE who should have full voting rights and undergo the same shortlisting and interview as all committee members (Norburn and Thomas, 2020).

A little less than a decade later, NICE decided to increase the committee lay member remit by having a lay member be part of the 'lead team' for each topic that was to be appraised (Norburn and Thomas, 2020). These lead teams consisted of three members of the committee who focused on one area each: cost-effectiveness, clinical effectiveness, and patient and carer evidence. This new role had the effect that lay members were both seen as an integral part of the team and became more informed and engaged in the topic and the evidence for consideration.

When NICE expanded its HTAs in 2009 to include assessments of medical technologies and diagnostic technologies, it was thus deemed necessary, alongside the two lay members on the committee, to recruit a patient (or carer) with topical knowledge of the technology or the condition being considered, who was a full member with voting rights on the committee. They were supported by the NICE PIP team and the committee team. This initiative was evaluated in 2010 with semi-structured interviews with both committee chairs and lay members, and in 2012 with a survey sent to all committee members. The conclusion from both evaluations was that the presence of the lay member on the lead team increased the visibility of patient evidence, all agreeing that this should become the new procedure. Lay members at NICE also help in developing HTA methods and processes as well as NICE's approach to patient involvement.

It is important to note that the PPI in diagnostics is different because there are specialist committee members instead of patient experts, who are recruited as extra lay members for a specific topic and participate in the decision-making for that evaluation, while still retaining the existing lay members who participate in all the diagnostics evaluations.

Patient experts in HTA

In addition to lay members whose role it is to take a generalist view in many topics, NICE decided early on that two persons (patient experts) should both submit a written statement and give testimony at committee meetings for HTAs on medicines, describing the views, perspectives and experiences of people affected by the technology or condition being considered. The experts are nominated and supported by patient organisations with additional support from NICE. The value of the patient expert contribution led NICE to involve patient experts in the field of Early Dialogues (Scientific Advice)[2] in 2014. The work with patient experts is continuously being evaluated, and the reported experiences of the patient experts have continued to improve, with 96% noting their experience as 'good' or 'excellent' in 2019–2020 (Norburn and Thomas, 2020).

In 2006, NICE decided to increase the input of patient evidence to the Interventional Procedures Guidance Programme, which assesses the efficacy and safety of procedures used for treatment or diagnosis. These procedures are usually new, posing different challenges, as knowledge is normally more limited than it is for medicines. Before this point, patient organisations, as well as individual patients and carers, had only been asked to comment on the draft guidance. This change meant they were asked to inform the committee's decision-making directly, by responding to an anonymous questionnaire. A summary report of the responses is put together by NICE and it is considered by the committee alongside the other evidence sources (Norburn and Thomas, 2020). For the assessment of medical technologies (this includes different types of medical devices) individual patient involvement is more flexible, but still aims to ensure the inclusion of patient survey data or patient expert input (NICE, 2017b).

---

2 Early Dialogues or Scientific advice is a fee-based advisory service offered by regulators and HTA agencies to developers of a range of health technologies, usually companies developing medicines.

NICE has also been an active partner in international HTA PPI work. It has, for example, contributed to the development of evidence submission templates for international patient organisations in medicines, non-medicines (MedTech) and diagnostics as members of the HTAi Patient and Citizen Involvement Interest Group (HTAi, 2013). It also actively participated in the development of the position statement on Patient Involvement produced by the International Network of Agencies for Health Technology Assessment (INAHTA) which was published in 2021 (INAHTA, 2021) and is an active member of the INAHTA Patient Engagement Learning Group. Such involvement enables staff members to learn from and embed international good practice.

The role of patient organisations in HTA

Throughout the history of NICE, patient organisations have contributed to the development of its working by commenting on NICE process and methods guides and collaborating to develop and improve how patients and carers are included. Patient organisations with an interest in the intervention or disease area being considered by NICE are invited to participate in the assessment. They can contribute in several different ways: the scoping of the HTA, involvement in consultations or workshops, by submitting patient evidence to HTA committees at NICE, by nominating patient experts to participate in committee meetings to give their individual perspectives and experiences, by giving their views on draft HTA guidance, by appealing final guidance for medicine HTAs, and lastly by supporting the final guidance to be put into practice (Norburn and Thomas, 2020: 4).

The importance of feedback in PPI has been highlighted at NICE. For example, committee members have been asked about their views on the impact of patient evidence for the Highly Specialised Technologies HTA programme (where treatments for very rare diseases are assessed). This has been used to give feedback to patient organisations when their evidence submission revealed new information or had an impact. Receiving such feedback helps patient organisations to know what areas to focus on in future submissions. Patient organisations are invited also to submit evidence in a template proforma, tailored to each topic, into the Interventional Procedures assessments (Norburn and Thomas, 2020). Patient involvement in NICE HTAs was further developed in 2019 when a core patient working group oversaw a project to 'capture a broad range of patient organizations' views, experiences, and suggestions for improvement through an event and survey' (Norburn and Thomas, 2020: 6).

Recent strengthening of public involvement at NICE

In 2021 PIP launched an expert panel to influence and inform NICE guidance and standards, to improve how NICE involves people who use services (including unpaid carers), and to use their experience to help others understand what NICE does and recommends. This expert panel provided an important opportunity to strengthen the community of individual patients who work with NICE. PIP aimed to recruit people who have a personal experience of using health or care services, are the carer or family member of a person using the services, are good at communicating, and have team-working skills and can use email and communicate online. The types of work undertaken by panel members include reviewing documents for accessibility and wording, providing quotes about experiences for NICE documents, providing feedback on public involvement, joining a group to work on a specific project, and raising awareness of how people can get involved with NICE.

The launch of the patient expert panel was followed by the launch of the Voluntary and Community Sector Forum in 2022 (NICE, 2023c). This brings together the organisations which want to inform and shape the work of NICE. It includes national bodies for people who use health and social care services, their families and carers, and the public. It also includes local Healthwatch organisations which represent patient voice in NHS and social care. NICE emphasised the importance of including a range of viewpoints and experiences and especially welcomed LGBTQIA+ people, ethnically diverse groups and people with disabilities.

In this section we have provided a detailed account of the way in which public involvement has developed at NICE. In the next section we reflect on the aspects of public involvement that need consolidation or strengthening in the future within the work of NICE.

A pivotal point for public and engagement involvement

As NICE marks 25 years of existence, we have reached a pivotal point for public involvement. There is much to celebrate in the achievements of the NICE Public Involvement Programme, including the building of a significant international reputation which has provided leadership and insight for other international agencies. However, past achievements in any organisation can never be interpreted as an indicator of future stability, as fiscal, political, and environmental pressures can impact on our desire for public voice at the heart of health and social care decision-making. With this in mind, we consider the areas where NICE needs to consolidate its work to ensure that it does not lose the gains it has achieved, in addition to areas where it needs to strengthen its public involvement.

Organisational factors

One of the factors that may be considered to have contributed to the continued embedding of involvement within NICE has been the longevity and stability of the team. Staff turnover in the Public Involvement Programme at NICE over 25 years has been relatively low. The Head of the Programme, Victoria Thomas, worked with the original Director at the start of NICE, Marcia Kelson, leading patient and public involvement for over 14 years until she left NICE in 2023. Many of the staff have also been with NICE for significant periods of time. Such organisational memory, alongside the significant knowledge accumulated about public involvement, has been an asset for NICE. The importance of that perspective on an international scale cannot be underestimated in helping others develop their involvement and engagement activities.

The evolution of public involvement

The College of Health provided the perspective of a critical friend in the early days of NICE, but the need for such a role reduced as involvement became increasingly embedded in practice. NICE evolved public involvement by aiming to follow best practice and adopting a continuous quality improvement approach, such as undertaking formal exit questionnaires with lay representatives to evaluate public involvement. Despite this focus on embedding, we would argue that there remains a sense of 'otherness' about involvement: important and integral, but somehow different from the remainder of NICE's work. Such 'otherness' needs attention to ensure public involvement becomes truly embedded in a way everyone understands. The reasons for this sense of 'otherness' could be many. They might include a lack of clarity about the values and specific aims of involvement, poor integration of involvement in the creation of concepts and methods used in research, or a limited understanding of the specific impact of involvement and where it can be targeted with greatest effect. Sometimes the 'otherness' may exist because the evidence base underpinning involvement is not drawn on as much as it could be, to ensure public involvement practice is valued and understood.

Values as drivers of activity

Public involvement can be underpinned and driven by a set of values that provide a deeper rationale for activity. While NICE does refer to specific involvement-focused values, there is a plan to develop more explicit values to underpin its involvement and engagement. To date, NICE has established an evidence-based conceptual framework around values such as legitimacy, fairness, equality and capacity building. NICE has developed values linked to HTA (Pinho-Gomes et al., 2022). This framework was mapped to current practice and a gap analysis undertaken. This work has informed the development of a draft strategy, drawing on the findings from a commissioned review of public involvement which is expected in 2024 (personal communication, Victoria Thomas, 2009). As this is not yet public, it is not possible to judge the way in which the identified values driving involvement in NICE have been represented in the future strategy. Recently, NICE also undertook a scoping review summarising the available evidence on principles, values, frameworks and strategies underpinning PPI by agencies involved in HTA and guideline development (Pinho-Gomes et al., 2022).

NICE could draw on the work of Gradinger et al. (2015), who provide a useful summary of values that underpin patient and public involvement. These include normative values that focus on empowerment, rights, accountability and transparency. They also identify substantive values that focus on the consequences of research (and so apply to NICE's research-based products) that involve patients and the public, enhancing the effectiveness, quality, relevance, reliability, and validity of research. Finally, Gradinger et al. identify process values concerned with elements such as partnership/equality, respect/trust, openness and honesty. It could be argued that many of these values provide a tacit underpinning for patient and public involvement at NICE, contributing to improving the quality and relevance of NICE products and outputs in ways that recognise the legitimacy of patient and public involvement. Our hope is that future activity would reflect the granularity offered by Gradinger et al. when describing values, not necessarily in a published strategy, but in NICE's own understanding of why and how it involves the public in its work.

The changing nature of evidence and knowledge

Patients and public contributors often identify forms of evidence or knowledge they regard as important in informing the development of guidance or in decision-making. For example, patient experiences of a condition or patient-important outcomes can provide vital evidence of the effectiveness, acceptability, and appropriateness of interventions. Such patient-based evidence (PBE) can complement the clinical and economic criteria of effectiveness and efficiency with a broader world view, reflecting the reality of peoples' lives.

While the wider research ecosystem has recognised the importance of qualitative evidence, NICE has drawn less on PBE to inform its work than it might have done, despite encouragement (Staniszewska and Werkö, 2017; Staniszewska and Werkö, 2021; Werkö and Staniszewska, 2021). In this pivotal point for public involvement, NICE could make a stronger statement about the value and use of PBE as a form of knowledge valued by patients and public contributors. For example, when it commissions an evidence review it could require three forms of evidence to be evaluated: clinical, economic and patient-based evidence. We would argue that this would reflect the original intent of Sackett et al.'s (1996) comment that the practice of evidence-based medicine means integrating individual clinical expertise (which includes a consideration of patients' preferences) with the best available external clinical evidence from systematic research. By best available clinical evidence they referred to clinically relevant research, often from the basic sciences of medicine, but 'especially from patient-centred clinical research' although the exact nature of this form of evidence was not specifically defined (Staniszewska and Werkö, 2021). This perspective is interesting, particularly as the etymology of the word 'evidence' is rooted in the concept of experience, relating to what is manifest and obvious (Upshur, 2001).

One example of this potential to extend the role of qualitative evidence is expressed by the work of Ziebland and colleagues (2014) who explored how the development of NICE quality standards could be informed by a secondary analysis of qualitative narrative interviews on patient experience. The inclusion of qualitative data on experiences and other aspects of care provides a more 'complete' view of evidence and offers the opportunity for a fuller evaluation of interventions and the creation by NICE of recommendations of relevance to patients, carers, service users and the public (Staniszewska and Werkö, 2021).

Developing the patient and public involvement and engagement evidence base

While NICE has developed the practice of patient and public involvement in its activities, the international evidence base has grown over the last few decades. For an organisation focused on the use of evidence, NICE is not explicitly guided by the public involvement evidence base to inform its practice, although it is guided by good public involvement practice. NICE has however contributed to the evidence base through peer-reviewed publication. For example, Scott et al. (2022) explored strategies for involving patients and the public in living guideline development panels during the pandemic. They identified eight strategies that both lay members and the staff and chairs mentioned as being important to effective involvement over time. These included technical training (such as PICO[3] and GRADE[4]), peer support, involvement in the scope, avoiding jargon, use of written personal statements about experiences,

3 PICO is a way to help structure a research question which is looking to find clinical information related to a specific patient group, intervention or therapy. PICO stands for:

P: Population/disease (i.e. age, gender, ethnicity, with a certain disorder)
I: Intervention or Variable of Interest (exposure to a disease, risk behavior, prognostic factor)
C: Comparison: (could be a placebo or "usual treatment" as in no disease, absence of risk factor, prognostic factor B)
O: Outcome: (risk of disease, accuracy of a diagnosis, rate of occurrence of adverse outcome)

4 GRADE (Grading of Recommendations, Assessment, Development, and Evaluations) is a transparent framework for developing and presenting summaries of evidence and provides a systematic approach for making clinical practice recommendations.

role description and involvement in dissemination and implementation. NICE's capacity to undertake public involvement research to inform practice should be included as a strategic research theme, or in collaboration with universities and organisations focused on developing the evidence base of public involvement.

There is also a potential role for patients and public contributors in the development or evolution of concepts, methods and processes used to create the evidence used by NICE, strengthening the way in which patients and the public shape health and social care evidence. NICE has taken important steps in this direction with work that has explored patient involvement in methods and process reviews (Rasburn, Livingstone and Scott, 2021). The specifics of the activity vary, but there is usually representation from PIP on any methods updates, and a consultation. This might also be supplemented by internal and external working groups, including voluntary and community groups. It might also require input from researchers who have a focus on developing patient-focused concepts and methods.

Prioritising evidence developed with patients, or the public could be an important next step for NICE. For example, by demanding that reviews of evidence always ask whether a primary research study had reported their public involvement, we could develop a much better understanding of the extent to which the evidence base underpinning NICE recommendations has been developed with patients and the public, and thus some assurance of quality in terms of focus, approach and relevance.

Innovation in implementation

NICE also has the potential to extend the public involvement role in its implementation work. The NICE Implementation Strategy (NICE, 2017a) aims for the organisation to 'both drive and enable the design and the effective delivery of services provided by the health and care system'. There is now a recognition that patients have an important role in helping to promote, disseminate and implement NICE guidance (Thomas, 2009). Nationally and internationally, there is a recognition that the production of guidance is not enough, and active ways of disseminating and implementing guidance are vital to achieve changes in health and social care practice and create patient and client or service user benefit. While implementation is represented by a large area of theoretically driven research, there has been much less focus on the patient and public role in implementation (Rycroft-Malone et al., 2016).

In establishing a NICE Implementation Strategy Group, NICE has considered the role of patients, carers and the public in implementation. As Thomas (2009) states:

Patients, carers and members of the public are in a unique position to identify when things are going well or badly in terms of the care they receive.

By involving them in getting NICE guidance into practice, organisations can help to ensure the recommendations from NICE are used in ways that are suitable, accessible, and easily available to the people they affect.

An important step in supporting patients and the public to be more involved in implementation is the provision of patient versions of guidance; although these have been discontinued, which limits public access to the detail of some of the guidance, which may impact on their capacity to be involved in implementation. There is still an 'information for the public' tab on each piece of guidance which summarises some core information and points people to other sources of support, such as the NHS website and patient organisations. PIP has worked closely with implementation activity, supporting public contributors to become involved in different ways. For example, it publishes a collection of activities undertaken by individual patients, members of the public and voluntary organisations that support the implementation of NICE guidance.

While NICE may not be best placed to provide publicly-facing health information, there are some important examples of patients and voluntary organisations promoting NICE guidance or supporting its dissemination and implementation for their membership. For example, the National Kidney Federation promotes many of the NICE guidelines at its annual conference and other meetings. In addition, NICE is a collaborator on an NIHR-funded study (PIPER) that is exploring the patient and public role in implementation and will create a toolkit to support patients and public contributors who want to develop a role or contribute to implementation. Such initiatives will strengthen the opportunities patients and public contributors have in changing health and social care practice.

Future development at NICE

NICE plans to review the public involvement programme. Importantly it states that it will develop and plan its future strategic relationships with patient, community and voluntary sector organisations including reconceptualising how stakeholders can contribute to its work more effectively (NICE, 2019/20). The Public Involvement team also wish to extend the use of deliberative approaches to public engagement to support debate about key issues, such as the ethical aspects of NICE's work. In addition, NICE intends to enhance the diversity of the lay members it works with. Internationally NICE wishes to strengthen its work with initiatives, such as EUPATI of which it is part of the founding and ongoing faculty. This provides an important opportunity for patient advocates to understand all aspects of medicines development. NICE plans to continue working closely with the Guidelines International Network (GIN), and INAHTA. In addition, NICE will continue its collaboration with other arm's length bodies through the People and Communities Forum, which is a coalition of patient and public involvement leads across all public bodies. The

Forum works together to support organisations to overcome some of the common challenges in public involvement. It provides an opportunity for organisations to share ideas, learning and successes. Importantly it will continue to support other organisations within health and social care in the UK, that want to develop their patient and public involvement strategies. The Forum is thus a key resource for the sector and an important source of legitimacy for those organisations.

The evidence that contributes to the work of NICE is increasingly likely to have patient and public involvement embedded within its creation. How NICE utilises this potential additional indicator of quality could send a powerful message to other agencies and organisations. It could be argued that NICE should consider privileging evidence that has been created through a high-quality patient and public involvement process. NICE could become more involved in studies that develop patient-important concepts in research which can then be used in creating the evidence which NICE draws upon. For example, NICE could be involved in or use research studies that develop frameworks to guide patient and public involvement in complex areas or offer important insights into patient-important concepts. We would also encourage NICE to embrace the concept of high-quality reporting of public involvement in research when it undertakes reviews of evidence. For example, it could routinely use the GRIPP2 guidance (Staniszewska et al., 2017) which is specifically focused on reporting public involvement in research, and the CHEERS 2022 guidance (Husereau et al., 2022) for health economic evaluation, which now includes two items specifically on public involvement. Finally, NICE has the potential to enhance the role of patients and public contributors in the implementation of health and social care evidence into practice. The role of patients, service users, carers, patient organisations and communities in using NICE evidence to create better health outcomes could be a key area for the future. This could also extend to more patient and public involvement in the de-implementation or disinvestment of interventions, identifying aspects of care patients and the public recognise as not being effective, acceptable, or appropriate.

Conclusion

The Public Involvement Programme has grown and strengthened over the last 25 years, enabled by strong, consistent leadership and with a team with relatively little staff turnover, who have been able to develop expertise in specific aspects of the work undertaken by NICE. The curation of this expertise places the team in a significant position of strength and will enable both NICE and the PIP team to further develop evidence-informed practice in the future. We would encourage NICE not to deplete that expertise as it is the foundation of high-quality practice. We also recognise the vital role NICE has played in offering leadership which has contributed to the legitimisation of patient and public involvement both nationally and internationally. Nationally, NICE has contributed to the growth of involvement and engagement across many health and social care agencies. Internationally, organisations have drawn on the exemplars often set by NICE in its patient and public involvement activity and have utilised this activity as a rationale for strengthening their own involvement activities.

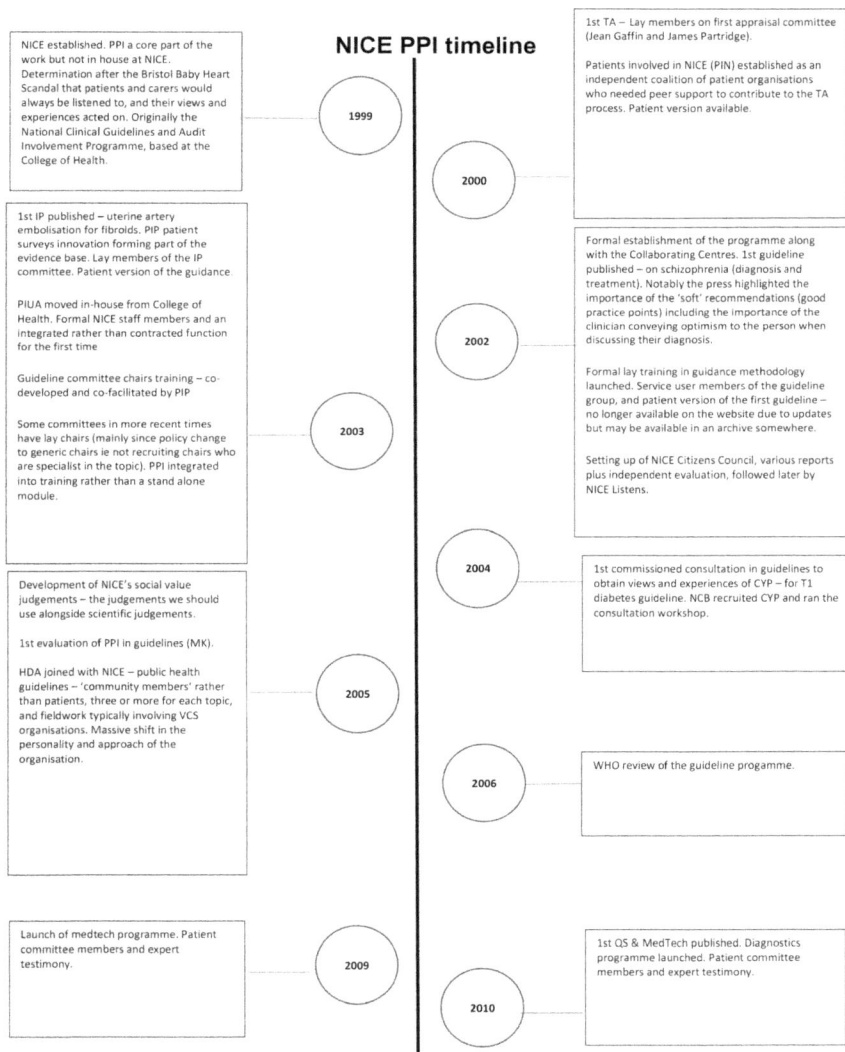

Figure 8.1 NICE PPI timeline

First diagnostics guidance published.

2011

Health & Social Care Act gives NICE new remit for social care – social care guidelines with culture of co-prodcution. Innovations e.g. adaptations, easy read and tailored support for people with learning disabilities on guideline committees (and workshops for recruiting people to the committee). Another innovation was young people's reference panel for Child Abuse and Neglect.
Patient experience guideline.

2012

1st HST guidance. Father of a patient with a haemolytic uraemic syndrome (HUS) came to a public Board meeting to thank it for the guidance that had saved his child. Shared Decision-making Collaborative.

2014

1st NICE patient decision aid (Atrial fibrillation – medicines tor reduce risk of stroke?) Suite of NICE PDAs.

2015

Antimicrobial resistance guidance. New approach to a suite of guidance on a shared topic – now becoming routine.

2017

2018

Social care experience.

Pancreatic Cancer UK wins shared learning award. First patient organisation to do so.

2019

2020

Covid-19 rapid guidelines – VCS organisational input despite incredibly short deadlines (and later lay member input). Long Covid joint publication with SIGN including patient information. PPI in virtual environment – work done to support participation with Zoom training, equipment support etc. Lay member training goes online. Lay member online training modules – 1st batch launched (2nd batch launched 2021).

PIP expert panel launched. Shared decision-making guideline published (a world first?) along with training resources etc.

Babies and children's experience guidance.

2021

2022

VCS Forum launch.

PPI framework development.

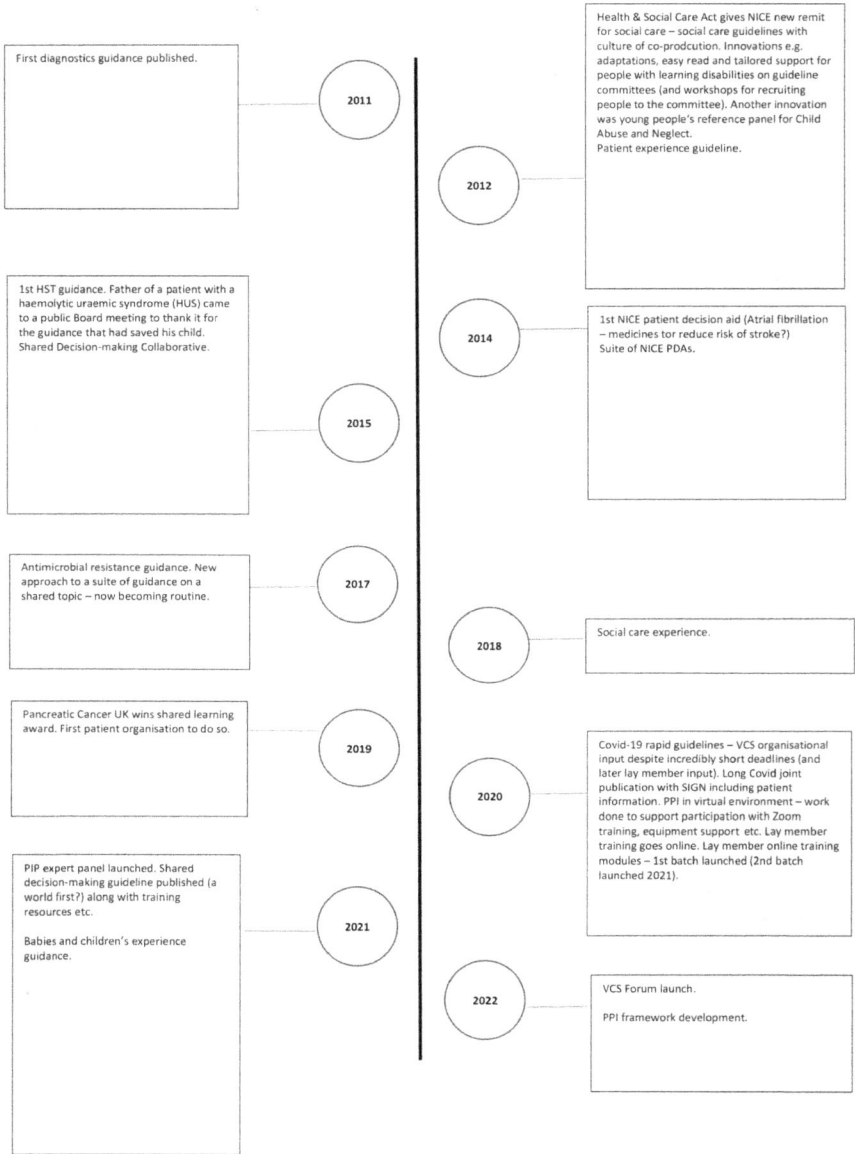

Figure 8.1 Continued

We must also consider the context in which NICE sits in relation to patient, community and voluntary organisations in the UK. These organisations have provided both strong challenge and strong support, and have helped ensure that focus remains on patient and public benefit, shaping core activities and ambitions. We would also urge NICE to work closely with funding agencies to help develop an agenda that supports the development of studies that add to our public involvement evidence base, that NICE can then draw upon to inform public involvement practice. While we recognise that such practice often sits alongside tacit practitioner knowledge, our perspective is that evidence will play an increasingly important role in enhancing future patient and public involvement, at NICE and elsewhere. It will provide a strengthening rationale in times where we expect resources for health and social care to diminish while patient need increases. In such a context, patient and public involvement and engagement will become even more important, and NICE will have a greater role as a beacon of excellence, both nationally and internationally.

References

Boivin, A., Currie, K., Fervers, B., Gracia, J., James, M., Marshall, C., Sakala, C., Sanger, S. et al. (2010) 'Patient and public in clinical guidelines: International experiences and future perspectives', *Quality and Safety in Health Care*, 19:e22.

Davies, C., Barnett, E. and Wetherell, M. (2006) *Citizens at the Centre: Deliberative Participation in Healthcare Decisions*. Bristol: Policy Press.

Davies, C., Barnett, E. and Wetherell, M. (2009) 'A citizens council in the making: dilemmas for citizens and their hosts', in Littlejohns, P. and Rawlins, M. (eds), *Patients, the Public and Priorities in Healthcare*. Oxford: Radcliffe, pp.129–38.

Dolan, P., Tsuchiya, A. and Wailoo, A. (2003) 'NICE's citizens council: What do we ask them, and how', *The Lancet*, 362(9387), pp.918–19.

Dyer, C. (2001) 'Bristol Inquiry condemns hospital's "club culture"', *British Medical Journal*, 323, p.181.

Gradinger, F., Britten, N., Wyatt, K., Frogatt, K., Gibson, A., Jacoby, A., Lobban, F., Mayes, D. et al. (2015) 'Values associated with public involvement in health and social care research: a narrative review', *Health Expectations*, 18(5), pp.661–75.

HTAi (Health Technology Assessment International) (2013) 'Resources and Materials: for patient groups and individual patients'. Available at: https://htai.org/patient-and-citizen-involvement/ (Accessed 30 March 2023).

Husereau, D., Drummond, M., Augustovski, F., de-Bekker-Grob, E. Briggs, A.H., Carswell, C., Caulley, L., Chaiyakunapruk, N. et al. (2022) 'Consolidated Health Economic Evaluation Reporting Standards 2022 (CHEERS 2022) statement: updated reporting guidance for health economic evaluations', *British Medical Journal*, 375:e067975.

INAHTA (International Network of Agencies for Health Technology Assessment) (2021) 'Position statement: patient involvement'. Available at: https://www.inahta.org/position-statements/ (Accessed 30 March 2023).

Kelson, M. (2005) 'The NICE Patient Involvement Unit', *Evidence-based Healthcare and Public Health*, 9(4), pp.304–07.

McCabe, C. and Round, J. (2019) 'Hard choices: reflections from the tomb of the unknown patient', *Healthcare Management Forum*, 32(6), pp.288–92.

NICE (2000) *Guidance on the Extraction of Wisdom Teeth*. TA1. London: NICE.

NICE (2010) *Uterine Artery Embolisation for Fibroids*. IPG367. London: NICE.

NICE (2011a) *The EOS 2D/3D Imaging System*. DG1. London: NICE.

NICE (2011b) *Service User Experience in Adult Mental Health: Improving the Experience of Care for People Using Adult NHS Mental Health Services*. CG136. London: NICE.

NICE (2012) *Patient Experience in Adult NHS Services: Improving the Experience of Care for People Using Adult NHS Services*. CG138. London: NICE.

NICE (2017a) 'The NICE Implementation Strategy: Principles and Approaches'. Available at: https://www.nice.org.uk/Media/Default/About/what-we-do/Into-practice/Help-Implement-NICE-guidance/Implementation-Strategy.pdf (Accessed 9 November 2023).

NICE (2017b) Medical Technologies Evaluation Programme Process Guide. PMG34. London: NICE.

NICE (2018) *People's Experience in Adult Social Care Services: Improving the Experience of Care and Support for People Using Adult Social Care Services*. NG86. London: NICE.

NICE (2019/20) *Public Involvement at NICE – Annual Report*. London: NICE.

NICE (2020) *Our Principles: The Principles that Guide the Development of NICE Guidance and Standards*. London: NICE.

NICE (2021a) *Babies, Children and Young People's Experience of Healthcare*. NG204. London: NICE.

NICE (2021b) *Shared Decision-making*. NG197. London: NICE.

NICE (2023a) 'NICE listens'. Available at: https://www.nice.org.uk/get-involved/nice-listens (Accessed 22 March 2023).

NICE (2023b) 'Patient and public involvement policy'. Available at: https://www.nice.org.uk/about/nice-communities/nice-and-the-public/public-involvement/public-involvement-programme/patient-public-involvement-policy (Accessed 22 March 2023).

NICE (2023c) 'Voluntary and Community Sector Forum'. Available at: www.nice.org.uk/about/nice-communities/nice-and-the-public/public-involvement/nice-voluntary-and-community-sector-forum (Accessed 22 March 2023).

NICE Citizens Council (2013) *What Aspects of Benefit, Cost and Need Should NICE Take into Account When Developing Social Care Guidance?* London: NICE.

Norburn, L. and Thomas, L. (2020) 'Expertise, experience, and excellence. Twenty years of patient involvement in health technology assessment at NICE: an evolving story', *International Journal of Technology Assessment in Health Care*, 37(10):e15, pp.1–7.

Pinho-Gomes A.C., Stone, J., Shaw, T., Heath, A., Cowl, J., Norburn, L., Thomas, V. and Scott, S. (2022) 'Values, principles, strategies, and frameworks underlying patient and public involvement in health technology assessment and guideline development: a scoping review', *International Journal of Technology Assessment in Health Care* 38(1):e46, pp.1–7.

PIPER (nd) 'Pathways to Implementation for Public Engagement in Research'. Available at: https://warwick.ac.uk/fac/sci/med/research/hscience/sssh/research/piper/ (Accessed 22 March 2023).

Rasburn, M., Livingstone, H., Scott, S.E. (2021) 'Strengthening patient outcome evidence in health technology assessment: a coproduction approach', *International Journal of Technology Assessment in Health Care*, 37:e12, pp.1–4.

Rycroft-Malone, J., Burton, C.R., Bucknall, T., Graham, I.D., Hutchinson, A.M. and Stacey, D. (2016) 'Collaboration and co-production of knowledge in healthcare: opportunities and challenges', *International Journal of Health Policy and Management*, 5(4), pp.221–23.

Sackett, D.L., Rosenberg, W.M.C., Muir Gray, J.A., Haynes, R.B. and Scott Richardson, W. (1996) 'Evidence based medicine; what it is and what it isn't', *British Medical Journal* 312, pp.71–72.

Scott, S.E., Chambers, E., Bayliss, K., Cowl, J., McFarlane, E., Rasburn, M., Tonkinson, M. and Wigmore, J. (2022) 'Strategies for involving patients and the public in living guideline development panels during the pandemic: a qualitative exploration'. Available at: https://www.researchgate.net/publication/357590079_Strategies_for_involving_patients_and_the_public_in_living_guideline_development_panels_during_a_pandemic_a_qualitative_evaluation#fullTextFileContent (Accessed 23 March 2023).

Staniszewska, S., Boardman, F., Gunn, L., Roberts, J., Clay, D., Seers, K., Brett, J. and Avital, L. (2014) 'The Warwick Patient Experiences Framework; patient-based evidence in clinical guidelines', *International Journal of Quality in Health Care*, 26(2), pp.151–57.

Staniszewska, S., Brett, J., Simera, I., Seers, K., Mockford, C., Goodlad, S., Altman, D.G., Moher, D. et al. (2017) 'GRIPP2 reporting checklist: tools to improve reporting of patient and public involvement in research', *British Medical Journal*, 358:j3453.

Staniszewska, S. and Werkö, S.S. (2017) 'Patient-based evidence in HTA', in Facey, K., Ploug Hansen, H., Single, A.N.V. (eds.) *Patient Involvement in Health Technology Assessment*. Adis: Singapore, pp.43–50.

Staniszewska, S. and Werkö, S.S. (2021) 'Mind the evidence gap: The use of patient-based evidence to create "complete HTA" in the twenty-first century', *International Journal of Technology Assessment in Health Care*, 37(1):e46, pp.1–7.

Street, J., Stafinski, T., Lopes, E. and Menon, D. (2020) 'Defining the role of the public in Health Technology Assessment (HTA) and HTA-informed decision-making processes', *International Journal of Technology Assessment in Health Care*, 36(2), pp.87–95.

Thomas, V. (2009) 'Patient and voluntary organisation support for implementing NICE Guidance', in Littlejohns, P. and Rawlins, M. (eds), *Patients, the Public and Priorities in Healthcare*. Oxford: Radcliffe, pp.57–64.

Upshur, R. (2001) 'The status of qualitative research as evidence', in Morse, J.M., Swanson, J.M. and Kuzel, A.J. (eds) *The Nature of Qualitative Evidence*. Thousand Oaks: Sage, pp.5–27.

Werkö, S.S. and Staniszewska, S. (2021) 'Patient and public involvement in Health Technology Assessment: a new dawn?', *International Journal of Technology Assessment in Health Care* 37(1):e54, pp.1–2.

WHO Europe (2006) *The Clinical Guideline Programme of the National Institute for Health and Clinical Excellence (NICE) A Review by the World Health Organization*. Geneva: WHO Europe.

Ziebland, S., Locock, L., Fitzpatrick, R., Stokes, T., Robert, G., O'Flynn, N., Bennert, K., Ryan, S. et al. (2014) *Informing the Development of NICE Quality Standards through a Secondary Analysis of Qualitative Narrative Interviews on Patient Experience*. Southampton: NIHR Journals Library (Health Services and Delivery Research, No. 2.45).

9 NICE and the law

Judicial oversight, juridification and legitimacy?

Keith Syrett

Introduction

NICE was born in the shadow of the law. The decision by the then Secretary of State for Health, Frank Dobson, to restrict prescription of the recently licensed drug sildenafil (Viagra) on the National Health Service (NHS) in 1998 prompted two court challenges by the manufacturer, Pfizer, in addition to generating substantial public and professional controversy. This 'first explicit, national rationing decision in the history of the NHS' (Klein and Williams, 2000: 25) proved to be such a legal and political hot potato that the establishment, shortly thereafter, of a body at arm's length from government with responsibility for issuing recommendations on the commissioning of new pharmaceutical and other technologies for use on the NHS might be seen as more than an instance of synchronicity (Chalkidou, 2009: 3; Wang, 2017: 665).

This chapter seeks to explore the interactions between NICE and the law over its 25-year history, focusing upon the process of judicial review which has formed the major mechanism through which legal scrutiny of the Institute has taken place, albeit that it is very infrequently used. The discussion is set against the background of the supposedly enhanced role for law in the modern 'regulatory state' (Majone, 1994), of which NICE may be said to be a manifestation.

The legal context

NICE's relationship with the courts should be understood against the backdrop of the broader question of judicial scrutiny of allocative decision-making in the NHS. At the time of the establishment of the Institute, an important trend in this form of legal activity was emerging. This arguably connected to the greater visibility of priority-setting occasioned by the establishment of the 'internal market' in 1990, which functioned to separate the commissioning and provision of health services (Syrett, 2004).

Previously, English courts had been inclined to treat challenges to the denial or restriction of access to healthcare treatments and services on grounds of

DOI: 10.4324/9781003501268-9

cost as matters which were fundamentally inappropriate for judicial resolution. However, commencing with the decision of Laws J in the *Cambridge HA* case in 1995 (*R v Cambridge Health Authority, ex parte B* [1995] 3 WLUK 164), they had demonstrated an increasing willingness to subject the *process* by which decisions on allocative priorities were reached to legal oversight. They accomplished this by obliging authorities to offer some degree of explanation for the choices made, and by ensuring that a mechanism existed through which an individual who had been denied access could demonstrate that they exceptionally merited it. Nonetheless, this role had important limitations. Notably, courts remained clear that the exercise of judgement by the initial decision-maker on the appropriate ordering of priorities and, relatedly, upon the matter of the overall affordability of a treatment or service, were immune from judicial intervention. For example, in the second of the cases involving Viagra, Simon Brown LJ stated that 'choosing between competing priorities as to where funds should be allocated, must be regarded as a political decision to be taken by Government' (*R (Pfizer) v Secretary of State for Health* [2002] EWCA Civ 1566, para 17).

At its inception, therefore, the likeliest avenue of successful legal challenge to NICE as an allocative decision-maker would appear to have been in relation to the fairness of its processes for appraisal of technologies or the development of clinical guidelines, as distinct from the substance of the recommendations which emerged from those processes. Furthermore, scope even for this limited form of judicial scrutiny was liable to be further reduced by the establishment of an appeals mechanism internal to NICE, which could serve to deflect challenges away from the courtroom.

Ostensibly, this might be regarded as a positive outcome. Diversion of time and resources into frequent episodes of litigation would clearly inhibit NICE's capacity to undertake its functions. Furthermore, legal challenges to the Institute would almost certainly provoke negative media coverage which might lead to a loss of confidence in NICE, and an unwillingness to engage with its work, on the part of stakeholders and the wider public.[1] From this perspective, then, legal intervention might be viewed as a problematic phenomenon, that is that 'the heavy involvement of the law in a public service is a measure of its failure rather than its success' (Commission on the NHS, 2000: 62).

However, an alternative viewpoint is possible. Law, including litigation, also has the capacity to play a facilitative role in so far as it can set standards for 'good administration' which can assist decision-makers in discharging their tasks in the public interest. In the particular context in which NICE operates, it has been argued that judicial oversight can contribute to assuring legitimacy for

---

1 This possibility is illustrated by the *Fraser* case, discussed further below, in which it was argued that four members of the NICE Guideline Development Group should not have been appointed because of conflicts of interest. The judge noted that the allegations which were made, although unfounded, could dissuade people from serving on similar groups in the future.

contentious allocative choices by ensuring that the process for making decisions complies with precepts of procedural justice (Syrett, 2007; Syrett, 2008). Specifically, judicial review can act to 'enforce' the other conditions of the 'accountability for reasonableness' model, to which NICE claimed adherence from an early stage of its existence (Rawlins, 2005). The evolving proceduralist orientation of the case-law, noted above, lends weight to the potential for the courts to act in this manner.

With this overall background established, I now turn to examine the various instances of legal challenge to NICE in detail.

The cases

Over the quarter-century of its existence, only five challenges to NICE have proceeded to a full hearing before the Administrative Court exercising its judicial review jurisdiction, with three of these subsequently being appealed. Of course, this does not represent the totality of judicial consideration of the Institute's work. Since an important aspect of NICE's role is to produce recommendations on best practice for the management of particular clinical conditions, NICE guidance is frequently germane to cases in which litigants argue that harm has been caused as a result of medical treatment which falls below the requisite standard of care, even though such guidance is expressly not intended to displace clinical judgement (see e.g. *Price v Cwm Taf University Health Board* [2019] EWHC 938 (QB)). In other instances, funding decisions made by commissioners of healthcare services might depart from NICE recommendations contained in clinical guidelines: although the latter are not mandatory, a court might regard any such variance as unlawful in the absence of a defensible justification for the commissioner's differing position (see e.g. *R (Rose) v Thanet Clinical Commissioning Group* [2014] EWHC 1182 (Admin)).

Such cases differ from those to be discussed here, however, in that NICE itself was not the subject of the legal challenge. By contrast, in the following instances, the claimants sought to argue that there were legally actionable deficiencies in the manner in which the Institute arrived at its recommendations. For clarity of exposition and ease of analysis, the cases have been categorised according to the identity of the primary claimant, that is: pharmaceutical company or individual. However, it should be noted that others, including various patient organisations, also participated in these cases as 'interested parties': that is, third parties who were directly affected by the claim.

(a) Challenges by pharmaceutical companies

The first judicial review challenge occurred in 2007, in relation to appraisal of the drug Aricept (donepezil) for the treatment of mild to moderate Alzheimer's Disease. Following a lengthy process, NICE had recommended that the product should only be made available on the NHS for sufferers of moderately severe dementia, with the consequence that access was excluded for some 60% of Alzheimer's patients. After an unsuccessful internal appeal, the manufacturer, together with other interested parties including the Alzheimer's Society, sought judicial review.

In the Administrative Court, arguments based upon both procedural unfairness and deficiencies in understanding and application of the evidence by NICE, which had led it to the determination that the drug was not cost-effective for the majority of patients, were dismissed. In relation to the latter point, the judge endorsed the decision of the internal appeal panel, observing that 'it is not possible to appeal against the Final Appraisal Determination simply because the appellant does not agree with it' (*Eisai Ltd. v NICE* [2007] EWHC 1941 (Admin), para 112). However, the claimants did succeed on a claim relating to non-discrimination in relation to the application of the guidance to those with learning difficulties and for whom English was not a first language.

In a subsequent appeal to the Court of Appeal, the claim of procedural unfairness was upheld. The Institute had not disclosed a fully executable version of the economic model produced during the appraisal process, so as to protect the intellectual property rights of those who had developed the model. This practice was found to be unlawful as it placed consultees 'at a significant disadvantage in challenging the reliability of the model. In that respect it limits their ability to make an intelligent response on something that is central to the appraisal process' (*R (Eisai Ltd.) v NICE* [2008] EWCA Civ 438, para 66).

The next challenge by a pharmaceutical manufacturer occurred in 2009. In *R (Servier Laboratories Ltd.) v NICE* [2009] EWHC 281 (Admin), the claimant company challenged guidance which limited NHS access to the drug Protelos (strontium ranelate) for treatment of osteoporosis in post-menopausal women to a defined group, on grounds of insufficiency of evidence of clinical and cost-effectiveness. As in *Eisai*, a mixture of points relating to the procedure adopted, the consideration and evaluation of evidence, and discrimination were raised.

The latter two arguments were dismissed. Holman J observed that 'the very reason for the existence of NICE is to make hard choices' (para 224) with which a court should be reluctant to interfere. However, the procedural challenge succeeded: here again, NICE had refused to disclose the economic model which had been used to inform its determination, but this time because of the existence of a confidentiality agreement. Nevertheless, the judge considered that NICE had breached its obligations in public law to 'take all reasonable steps to seek permission . . . to release the data' in the interests of transparency (para 139).

The manufacturer appealed solely on the issue relating to consideration of data. It argued that NICE had failed to give adequate reasons for rejection of a particular study which, it was claimed, demonstrated the clinical efficacy of the drug; and that, even if those reasons had been adequately expressed, the rejection of the data and the consequent assessment of efficacy was not a position which could rationally have been taken. In this instance, the claim succeeded. Smith LJ concluded that the rejection of particular data by the Institute was 'inadequately explained. I cannot tell what its reasons are and I accept Servier's claim that it cannot either' (*Servier Laboratories Ltd. v NICE* [2010] EWCA Civ 346, para 45). Moreover, the judge made observations (albeit not legally binding) to the effect that NICE's departure from conclusions reached by the European Medicines Agency (EMA) might be unlawful in the absence of reasons for such departure. This position was endorsed by Pill LJ: 'it is not suggested that NICE are bound by EMA's decision or its reasoning but the appellants are entitled to expect any decision against them to be properly reasoned, especially when it is contrary to the reasoned decision of an equally eminent body' (para 62).

In the third case, the pharmaceutical manufacturer was less successful. *Bristol-Myers Squibb Pharmaceuticals Ltd. v NICE* [2009] EWHC 2722 (Admin) concerned appraisal of the drug abatacept for treatment of rheumatoid arthritis. As in the previous cases, one of the areas of challenge related to release of the economic model which underpinned the determination of cost-effectiveness. In this instance, the manufacturer contended that NICE had unfairly failed to release a fully executable form of the manufacturer's own economic model which had been modified during the appraisal process by the independent group appointed to review the evidence, the consequence being that it was 'unable to make effectively informed representations on the criticisms of its own costings by analysing the computations made by [the group] and responding to them' (para 22). Although Blake J emphasised that NICE was bound to observe principles of fairness in its decision-making process, he considered that these had not been breached in this case. This was because there had been disclosure of the variations made to the model during the consultation process which would have enabled the manufacturer, unlike Eisai, to run its own model based upon the alternative figures; consequently it had had the opportunity to make informed and effective representations during the appraisal process.

A further ground of challenge related to compliance with EU law, specifically the Transparency Directive (Council Directive 89/105 EEC), which requires publication and communication to the European Commission of those criteria which are taken into account in reaching determinations on whether medicinal products are included in, or excluded from, a national health system. The UK government had sought to comply with this Directive following the first of the cases concerning Viagra; the specified criteria included a statement that products might be excluded where the forecast aggregate cost to the NHS could not be justified in light of the statutory duties relating to provision of a comprehensive health service and the setting of priorities for expenditure of resources. It was argued that this statement, which concerned affordability, was now insufficient given the development by NICE of a 'more sophisticated model for assessing cost-effectiveness' (para 42). This was rejected by the court, which noted that cost-effectiveness was a subset of affordability rather than a distinct matter, and that the modest degree of transparency required by the Directive did not necessitate communication of the particular means by which the criterion of affordability might be assessed and applied.

(b) Challenges by individuals

The challenge in *R (Fraser) v NICE* [2009] EWHC 452 (Admin) concerned the making of a clinical guideline on provision of care for sufferers of chronic fatigue syndrome/myalgic encephalomyelitis. This had recommended a variety of approaches to treatment for those with mild or moderate forms of the condition, including cognitive behavioural therapy and/or graded exercise therapy, as being interventions for which there was clearest research evidence of benefit. The guideline was opposed by claimants who considered that its apparent preference for a psycho-social approach to the nature, cause and treatment of the condition was misplaced; they believed that these forms of treatment were ineffectual and potentially harmful to certain sufferers.

The claimants advanced two legal arguments. The first was that the guideline had placed too much weight on a review and evaluation of relevant randomised controlled and other trials which NICE had itself indicated (in the draft consultation guideline) that it considered not to be an adequate foundation of definitive guidelines with, contrastingly, insufficient weight to the experience of patients; and that it had overlooked the risks of cognitive behavioural and graded exercise therapies. This argument was briskly rejected by the court, which noted that it was a matter for the Institute's Guideline Development Group to determine what weight to attach to evidence: 'decisions of fact are for those entrusted to make those decisions' (para 64). The second argument was that certain members of the Group had a predetermination ('apparent bias') in favour of the psycho-social approach to treatment, this being in violation of legal principles of procedural fairness. This also received little judicial support. Simon J noted that all the impugned members had open minds as to the evidence, and commended NICE for its 'proper and effective system . . . to ensure that, so far as possible, there was no conflict of interest and duty among the membership of the Guideline Development Group' (para 109).

The second challenge in this category concerned the process adopted for technology appraisal of the product Kuvan (sapropterin dihydrochloride) as a treatment for the condition phenylketonuria. The argument in *R (Cotter) v NICE* [2020] EWHC 435 (Admin) was that the selection by the Institute of the standard appraisal process rather than the highly specialised technology process was unlawful in that it was based upon a misunderstanding and misreading of its own guidance on the application of the latter process. From the claimant's perspective, the matter was of considerable significance because (it was contended), the prospects of a positive recommendation for Kuvan were much higher under the highly specialised technology process, given a higher cost-effectiveness threshold of £100,000 per QALY as distinct from £20,000 to £30,000 per QALY.

The claimant's arguments were rejected by the Administrative Court. Cavanagh J considered the various criteria for the use of the highly specialised technology process which NICE had determined not to be satisfied in the case of Kuvan, and ruled that the Institute had not misunderstood or misapplied any of these. An appeal to the Court of Appeal was similarly unsuccessful ([2020] EWCA Civ 1037), although the court did suggest that the criteria for application of the highly specialised technology process should be set out in plain language 'which could be readily understood by patients and those caring for them' (para 83).

Analysing the case law

An initial, albeit perhaps unsurprising, observation which might be made about these cases is that pharmaceutical manufacturers have enjoyed greater success in pursuing legal claims against NICE than individuals. In only one instance, *Bristol-Myers Squibb*, did none of the grounds advanced on behalf of the company succeed; by contrast, not a single argument advanced in the cases brought by individuals convinced a judge to rule in their favour. Of course, in principle, the identity of the claimant in a judicial review action should make no difference to the application of legal norms. The likely explanation for the difference in outcome, therefore, lies in contextual factors: it seems plausible to assume that the greater resources available to pharmaceutical manufacturers enabled the development of more persuasive legal arguments, advanced by superior teams of lawyers.

Turning to the reasoning of the judges in these cases, it is helpful first of all to distinguish between arguments based upon deficiencies in the process of decision-making, and those which relate more directly to the content, or substance, of the guidance or guideline. As noted earlier in this chapter, the evolving jurisprudence on review of priority-setting in healthcare manifested a divergence between these two aspects: judges were much more willing to overturn decisions on procedural grounds than to 'second-guess' the judgment of the original decision-maker on the weighing of evidence and the resultant establishment of allocative priorities. This bifurcation in the level of judicial scrutiny is reflective of the law of judicial review in general. Substantive review is problematic because it violates principles of the separation of powers and parliamentary sovereignty: it is the original decision-maker which has been conferred with authority by Parliament (generally, by means of legislation) to apply its expertise in reaching the allocative choice in question, rather than a judiciary which lacks comparable expertise. Accordingly, review of the content of administrative decisions was traditionally only permissible in extreme cases where the choice made was 'so outrageous in its defiance of logic or of accepted moral standards that no sensible person who had applied his mind to the question to be decided could have arrived at it' (*CCSU v Minister for the Civil Service* [1983] UKHL 6).

A close reading of these cases, however, suggests that the differentiation between acceptable procedural review and unacceptable review of substance manifests a greater degree of nuance than is often assumed. Rather, it is possible to analyse the bases of review adopted by the courts as being located on a continuum which runs from 'pure process' to 'pure substance', with a further category between these poles.

(a) 'Pure process' review: transparency and bias

This was the most fruitful of the arguments advanced by the claimants in these cases. Each of the cases brought by pharmaceutical manufacturers included an argument that the NICE appraisal process lacked a degree of transparency in relation to release of the economic model which informed the Institute's recommendations on cost-effectiveness; and this ground was successful in two of these cases. Correspondingly, the judges sought to emphasise the considerable significance of transparency, and procedural fairness more generally, to the lawfulness of Institute decision-making. For example in the High Court decision in *Servier*, Holman J stated that 'NICE is always under a duty and imperative of transparency and fairness' (para 115) and observed that it must 'keep firmly in mind the high importance of fairness and transparency' (para 123).

There was widespread judicial acknowledgment of the efforts that NICE had made in this regard: for example, in the Court of Appeal decision in *Eisai*, it was commended for the fact that there was 'already a remarkable degree of disclosure and of transparency in the consultation process' (para 66). Paradoxically, however, these high standards created a space for judicial intervention: hence, the court continued by saying that the commitment to transparency 'cuts both ways because it also serves to underline the nature and importance of the exercise being carried out. The refusal to release the fully executable model stands out as the one exception to the principle of openness and transparency that NICE has acknowledged as appropriate in this context'. Similarly, in *Servier*, Holman J held that while exceptionally it might be permissible to give undertakings as to confidentiality in order to ensure the quality and robustness of the appraisal process, the high importance attached to transparency placed NICE 'under some duty to "press"', that is to 'particularly strive to seek permission to disclose the economic model and/or the data contained therein' (paras 121, 123).

As articulated in these cases, transparency in decision-making was not primarily accorded value in and of itself. Rather, its importance resided in its connection to meaningful participation in the appraisal process. Hence, the Court of Appeal in *Eisai* noted that the failure to release a fully executable version of the economic model disadvantaged the manufacturer and other consultees because it limited their 'ability to make an intelligent response on something that is central to the appraisal process' (para 66); while the High Court in *Servier* ruled that disclosure of the model was necessary to 'permit all consultees to make further submissions or representations in response to that disclosure' (para 230). This rationale for transparency in the appraisal process serves to explain the different conclusion reached in *Bristol-Myers Squibb*, since in this instance the failure to make full disclosure had not inhibited the capacity of the manufacturer to make representations during the consultation process.

Obligations of procedural fairness in the law of judicial review have traditionally been divided into two subcategories: the right to a fair hearing – which encompasses the arguments detailed above, since deficiencies in transparency inhibited the ability of the manufacturers adequately to 'state their case' – and the right to an independent and impartial decision-maker. The latter was at issue in *Fraser*, where the claimant maintained that certain members of the Guideline Development Group were predisposed towards a certain form of treatment. While this argument did not succeed, it should be noted that the court did not dismiss it out of hand; rather, the judge carefully examined the evidence advanced against each of the individuals in question before concluding in NICE's favour. However, a claim of predisposition was in any case likely to be difficult to make out given that (as the court noted) it carried costs for the Institute's decision-making process: that is, that it might deter experts from assisting NICE in its guideline development work in the future. By contrast, the only discernible cost of disclosure of the economic model in the manufacturer cases was that it worked against obligations of confidentiality which underpinned the quality and robustness of the appraisal process; however, since the affected individual in the *Servier* case had indicated that he was willing to waive the undertaking as to confidentiality to permit release of the fully executable model to consultees ([2009] EWHC 281 (Admin), para 142), this was not in practice problematic.

(b) *'Mixed procedural and substantive' review: reason-giving*

The 'accountability for reasonableness' model to which NICE sought to adhere, especially in the early period of its existence, is widely viewed as a framework of procedural justice; the Institute referred to it as such in its set of principles for the consideration of social values in the development of guidance (NICE, 2008). The first of the four conditions of the model, 'publicity', speaks to the transparency of decision-making as discussed in the preceding subsection. However, the second condition, 'relevance', summarised in the same document as meaning that 'the grounds for reaching decisions must be ones that fair-minded people would agree are relevant in the particular context' (ibid.) serves to rule in and rule out certain criteria on the basis that some are fairer than others. It has been argued that this is clearly a substantive requirement (Rid, 2009).

The two conditions are not, however, entirely separable from one another. This is again made apparent in *Social Value Judgements*, which describes the 'publicity' condition as meaning that 'both the decisions made about limits on the allocation of resources, *and the grounds for reaching them*, must be made public' (NICE, 2008: emphasis added). The requirement to be transparent about the criteria upon which decisions are made – in the jargon of judicial review, an obligation to give reasons for decisions – opens up the possibility that a decision may be ruled unlawful in the absence of sufficient justification of the bases upon which it is premised, the implication being that the decision may not have been rationally grounded upon the evidence which was available. As Shapiro (1992) observes, albeit in an American context, this is closer to review of substance than of procedure.

This form of review was at play in two of the decisions involving pharmaceutical manufacturers, with differing outcomes. In *Bristol-Myers Squibb*, the failure to present more detailed criteria of cost-effectiveness to the European Commission under the terms of the 'Transparency Directive' was not unlawful. It is notable, however, that in this case the High Court was bound by precedent emanating from the Court of Appeal decision in the second of the cases concerning Viagra, in which Buxton LJ had indicated that the degree of explanation of the relevant criteria required by the Directive was 'fairly modest' (*R (Pfizer Ltd. v Secretary of State for Health* [2002] EWCA Civ 1566, para 27).

By contrast, in the Court of Appeal decision in *Servier*, the absence of reasoned explanation for NICE's rejection of a post hoc subgroup analysis which was central to the drug manufacturer's case for clinical effectiveness was the main basis for the court's ruling against the Institute. The juxtaposition of procedural and substantive grounds for judicial intervention – the latter expressed by means of the concept of 'irrationality' – is clearly visible in this judgment. The fact that the rejection was 'inadequately explained' (para 45) led Smith LJ to express 'grave doubts about [the] rationality' of the recommendation made by NICE (para 46). She noted that:

> on the face of the decision as explained in the Final Appraisal Determination, the only reason given for the rejection of the data is that it came from a post hoc subgroup. The implication is that that class of scientific evidence is inherently unreliable. In my view, that reason *simpliciter* is not rational. The evidence of NICE itself is to the effect that such data may in some circumstances be acceptable and reliable. Therefore, if such data is to be rejected, the reason for rejection must relate to the particular study. If the evidence is considered to be weak, NICE must explain why it is of that view (para 48).

Similar reasoning underpinned the court's observations that the Institute's departure from the position taken by the European Medicines Agency on the subgroup data required justification: 'I would expect to see some reason given for NICE reaching a different view from a body of similar standing' (para 52).

(c) Substantive review: questions of judgement

These cases also demonstrate that there are a range of matters with which courts are reluctant to interfere, on the basis that they are issues which require the exercise of expert judgement by the Institute. These are instances in which the judiciary expresses 'deference' to NICE, a term which connotes that the court pays respect to its decisions by according substantial weight to them. The consequence of this approach is to make it highly unlikely that NICE will be found to have acted unlawfully in regard to these matters.

Perhaps the clearest expression of this position is the statement of Holman J in the *Servier* case in the High Court: 'it is important to stress at the outset that NICE is the specialist, expert body charged with making appraisals and decisions of this type. The court is not. I have neither the right, nor still less the expertise, to review the decisions as to their substance' (para 6). From this, it is possible to discern that there are two rationales for judicial deference which stem from deficiencies in judicial competence (Syrett, 2007). Courts lack *institutional competence* in that judges do not possess the requisite knowledge and understanding to carry out the tasks of technology appraisal and guideline development: as Pill LJ stated in the Court of Appeal decision in the same case, 'judgements on medical and scientific matters are required and the court should be more deferential than in other contexts when considering decisions taken' (para 58). Additionally, they lack *constitutional competence* in so far as it is NICE, not the judiciary, which has been directed by government to undertake these tasks.

Accordingly, so long as proper justification is put forward, the courts will not challenge the evaluation of evidence by NICE, nor the recommendations which it reaches on the basis of that analysis (unless the latter violates specific legal obligations which exist under non-discrimination legislation, as was the case in *Eisai*). For example, in *Fraser*, Simon J was clear that 'it was for the Guideline Development Group to decide what weight to attach to evidence' (para 64), while in the High Court in *Eisai*, Dobbs J observed that 'the court has no part to play in adjudicating between the rival merits of the arguments of the experts' (para 111).

In *Cotter*, it became apparent that this deferential approach extended also to interpretation of criteria governing the choice of appraisal process: that which counsel for NICE described as the 'routeing decision' ([2020] EWCA Civ 1037, [11]). While the criteria did not give rise to 'highly technical scientific questions', they did 'raise questions of degree which someone who is familiar with the approach to, and treatment of, rare and very rare conditions in the NHS will be better placed than a judge to answer' ([2020] EWHC 435 (Admin), para 68). Hence, while a court should not simply accept NICE's understandings of the meaning of the criteria without question, these should nonetheless be 'given proper respect', it being 'appropriate to bear in mind that this decision involved issues of judgement and was vested in a group of people with particular experience and expertise to take it' (ibid.: para 69).

Setting the case law in context: juridification in the regulatory state?

The establishment of NICE in 1999 can be seen as an illustration of how contemporary governance in the United Kingdom has gravitated towards the 'regulatory state' model which, during the greater part of the twentieth century, was rather 'one of the distinctive features of American exceptionalism' (Levi-Faur and Gilad, 2004: 105). Creation of autonomous regulatory agencies, such as the Institute, is a central feature of this model: its role in guiding and structuring NHS care stands in contrast to the professional self-regulation which had largely predominated within the Service since 1948 (Newdick, 2014), and which could be viewed as a manifestation of 'club government' (Moran, 2003: 4; Brown and Calnan, 2013: 65).

This traditional approach to regulatory governance had little to do with the law. Moran (2003: 68) explains:

> Self-regulation in Britain has also traditionally been distinguished by another kind of informality: the British have been reluctant to codify rules in detail, and correspondingly reliant on trust and implicit understandings. Finally, self-regulation in Britain has taken an unusual legal form: private associations, often entirely unknown to the law, have been central to many of the most important systems of self-regulation; and the law itself has historically played no role, or only a residual one, in the life of self-regulatory systems ... A summary way to express all this is as follows. Self-regulation in the British system can be described in terms of three variables: the degree to which systems are institutionalized, that is, are built around specialized institutions of control; the degree to which they codify their rules, that is, make them explicit rather than simply relying on tacit understandings; and the degree to which substantive rules and procedures are juridified, that is, are expressed in the language of the law and integrated with the wider legal system. The language of institutionalization, codification, and juridification revealingly isolates what has historically been comparatively distinctive about self-regulation in Britain: low levels of institutionalization, codification, and juridification have marked the system.

By contrast, 'the regulatory state is a juridified state' (Moran, 2000: 12). Moran (2003: 68) defines juridification as 'signify[ing] the rise of legal rules, legal reasoning, and resort to legal institutions to administer regulation': it encompasses processes such as the regulation of increasing numbers of activities through law, the resolution of increasing numbers of conflicts by or with reference to law, increased power accorded to lawyers and the legal system, and a more adversarial approach to relationships with stakeholders (Blichner and Molander, 2008; Moran, 2000).

Undoubtedly, the regulatory state thesis can make a useful contribution to an understanding of NICE and its work. For example, we may see the very establishment of the Institute as an example of the 'institutionalization' of certain standards of care and modes of allocative decision-making in the NHS which were previously matters largely determined by those working within the Service. Furthermore, we might view the detailed documentation of methodologies for its work and processes for stakeholder involvement, as well as the outputs which eventuate – clinical guidelines and technology appraisal guidance – as illustrative of a tendency towards 'codification'. However, this chapter's central concern with legal relations renders the 'juridification' dimension of Moran's tripartite framework of greatest interest.

From one perspective, the scarcity of legal challenges to NICE's work over the past quarter-century would seem to contradict claims of juridification. There is little evidence of an increasing level of conflict between the Institute and pharmaceutical companies, patient groups or affected individuals which has been mediated through legal mechanisms: in fact, the trend is rather for the *de-escalation* of conflict and adversarial relations expressed through law, with only one legal challenge (*Cotter*) having been commenced subsequent to the first decade of NICE's existence.

However, such a conclusion would seem to amount to too restrictive a reading of the concept of juridification. This should be understood as a broader matter than *judicialisation*, which refers to an increase in judicial power, especially through encroachment upon fields which are not usually regarded as sitting within the province of the judiciary. There is certainly little evidence of the occurrence of the latter phenomenon in relation to NICE. Not only have there been very few legal cases overall, but – as discussed above – even in instances where litigation has taken place, judges frequently demonstrate considerable reluctance to intrude upon areas which fall within the scope of NICE's expertise.

Instead, a broader understanding of juridification as a process of framing through a legal lens (Blichner and Molander, 2008), that is a situation in which matters come to be 'expressed in the language of the law and integrated with the wider legal system' (Moran, 2003: 68), has much greater validity as a descriptor of NICE's relations and activities. In this light, it is important to note that the Institute's internal technology appraisal appeals process is designed, in essence, to replicate the judicial review jurisdiction. This is so in two ways. First, the bases of appeal, that NICE has acted unfairly or in excess of power, and/or has issued a recommendation which is unreasonable in light of the evidence presented to it, mirror the standard grounds of judicial review (respectively, procedural impropriety, illegality and irrationality: see *CCSU v Minister for the Civil Service* [1984] UKHL 9). Secondly, the process mimics the independence of the courtroom, with a majority of Appeals Panel members being independent of NICE and an external chair; the process is managed by the corporate office at NICE to avoid any conflict of interest with those involved with development of the guidance which is at issue. It is notable that this internal mechanism has been utilised much more frequently than the judicial review process, with over 100 cases heard by the Appeals Panel between 2000 and 2022. This demonstrates an adversarial dimension to the work of NICE which is consistent with the juridification thesis, but which is not adequately captured by a consideration of the instances of litigation with which it has been involved.

Additionally, the changing normative bases upon which NICE rests its decision-making may be viewed as consistent with juridification. The long-standing commitment to 'accountability for reasonableness', noted above, represents engagement with a model of procedural justice which, as the present author has argued elsewhere, corresponds closely to a particular vision of the role of public law, and the judicial review jurisdiction in particular (Syrett, 2007; Syrett, 2008). More recently, NICE appears to have modified its decisional approach to technology appraisal. Charlton (2020: 196) observes that 'NICE's documented approach has become increasingly standardised, specified and detailed: that is, it has become more formalised', with a number of 'decision-rules' emerging, which limit scope for the exercise of value judgements by NICE committees. The trend to make decisions with reference to rules (albeit, not *legal* rules) is a clear instance of juridification in the broader sense of the term.

Revisiting the 'legitimacy problem'

Situating NICE as a component of the regulatory state carries further implications for analysis of its relations with the legal system. The originator of the model, Giandomenico Majone – following John Locke – argues that delegation of powers to independent agencies (such as the Institute) creates problems of legitimacy (Majone, 1999: 7; see also Brown and Calnan, 2013). This reinforces the particular problem identified by Norman Daniels and James Sabin (2008) that confronts institutions making priority-setting choices in healthcare: that such decisions (and, by extension, the bodies which make them) may struggle to attain public acceptability in light of the absence of an agreed ethical consensus on the substantive bases on which these might be made.

In earlier work (Syrett, 2002), and as noted briefly above, I argued that law, and especially judicial review, carried the potential to make a positive contribution to addressing problems of legitimacy which NICE might face. It seems appropriate now, some two decades later, to conclude this discussion of the interaction between the Institute and the legal system by reconsidering this evaluation.

Taken on their own, the court cases correspond broadly with the proceduralist orientation of the earlier jurisprudence on allocative decision-making which was previously outlined. The impact of these cases is to reinforce NICE's commitment to procedural justice through close judicial oversight of the transparency of its processes. This has the related consequence that stakeholders (mainly, pharmaceutical manufacturers) are able to participate more meaningfully in that they are 'able to understand what is at issue, to present evidence and arguments and to respond to or rebut opposing arguments' (Syrett, 2011: 483). This judicial activity may be set alongside a well-used and independent internal appeals process, which additionally permits the revisiting and revision of decisions in light of further evidence. In this manner, two of the four conditions of 'accountability for reasonableness' ('publicity' and 'appeals/revision') would appear to be fulfilled. Furthermore, although it has been infrequently utilised, the cases show that the judicial review jurisdiction can act as a form of external oversight of compliance with these conditions, thus meeting the third of the four criteria specified in the original model, 'enforcement/regulation'.

It is in respect of the remaining condition of the model, 'relevance', that legal oversight appears incomplete. Leaving aside very specific obligations deriving from anti-discrimination laws, the strong tendency of judges to defer to NICE's expertise – with one partial exception, the appeal decision in *Servier* – means that there is no genuine judicial scrutiny of the substantive bases upon which NICE rests its specific recommendations, or more broadly, of its overall approach to allocative decision-making (for example, the use of a QALY threshold in technology appraisals). This is an entirely comprehensible stance given the relative lack of institutional and constitutional competence of the judiciary; furthermore, it is consistent with the traditionally limited ambit of judicial review. However, it carries the additional consequence that accountability through legal process is not in itself sufficient to redress the deficit in democratic legitimacy which arises from NICE's status as an independent agency functioning within the regulatory state. This is a point underlined by McPherson and Sunkin (2020: 231), who argue that 'NICE appears largely free from legal accountability because courts tend to defer to experts; Parliament has given NICE authority to decide among the various scientific arguments'.

Turning from the court cases to juridification in its broader sense, a mixed picture also presents itself. On the one hand, as Charlton (2020: 209) observes, the trend towards standardisation, documentation and formalisation 'has the potential to enhance fairness if it acts to increase the consistency of decision-making across similar cases': since achieving consistency is one of the goals of the 'publicity' condition of 'accountability for reasonableness', this can enhance legitimacy. Moreover, the most recent formal statement of the Institute's principles for development of its standards and guidance (NICE 2020) continues to foreground transparency, demonstrating that this value 'remains central to its conception of procedural justice' (Charlton, 2022: 130). This suggests a continued commitment to 'accountability for reasonableness', notwithstanding that this model is not explicitly referenced in the document.

However, Charlton's work also identifies important ways in which formalisation has impeded, rather than enhanced, the pursuit of legitimacy. She notes that NICE has failed to offer justification of the criteria upon which the emerging decision-rules are based; that the existence of such rules limits the scope for deliberation which 'accountability for reasonableness' is intended to facilitate; and that those value judgements which remain embedded in the decisional process are also not fully explained. Overall, she detects an 'apparent reluctance to provide a full account of the varied substantive criteria now embedded across its methods' (Charlton, 2022: 135), concluding that its recent statement of decisional principles

> grounds . . . claims for fairness and legitimacy almost entirely on the Institute's procedural strengths, eschewing acknowledgement of the more contentious substantive considerations that have recently become embedded within its methods . . . in attempting primarily to avoid rather than address underlying questions about these judgements, [the document] undermines the transparency on which NICE's notion of procedural justice relies (ibid.: 135–6).

Conclusion

Perhaps surprisingly, given the conditions which surrounded its creation and the highly controversial work which it undertakes, NICE has relatively rarely engaged with the legal system in a formal manner, through litigation. Nevertheless, as an archetype of the regulatory state, the Institute – increasingly – exhibits various characteristics of juridification which demonstrate that the influence of legal norms and thinking extends beyond the courtroom.

The question of legitimacy, which is of central concern to legal scholarship (Prosser, 1982; Longley, 1993), has been the subject of critical analysis from the earliest days of the Institute (Syrett, 2002). A quarter of a century on, and notwithstanding certain continuing deficiencies of the type identified by Charlton, NICE would seem to have attained a degree of acceptance and respect as a decision-maker which would indicate that its legitimacy has largely been secured. If that is so, the argument presented here would suggest that the contribution of law to this achievement is more nuanced than might have been anticipated.

References

Blichner, L. and Molander, A. (2008) 'Mapping juridification', *European Law Journal*, 14(1), pp.36–54.

Brown, P. and Calnan, M. (2013) 'NICE technology appraisals: working with multiple levels of uncertainty and the potential for bias', *Medicine, Health Care and Philosophy*, 16(2), pp.281–93.

Chalkidou, K. (2009) 'Comparative effectiveness review within the UK's National Institute for Health and Clinical Excellence', *Issue Brief (Commonwealth Fund)*, 59, pp.1–12.

Charlton, V. (2020) 'NICE and fair? Health technology assessment policy under the UK's National Institute for Health and Care Excellence, 1999–2018', *Health Care Analysis*, 28(3), pp.193–227.

Charlton, V. (2022) 'Justice, transparency and the guiding principles of the UK's National Institute for Health and Care Excellence', *Health Care Analysis*, 30(2), pp.115–45.

Commission on the NHS, chaired by Will Hutton. (2000) *New Life for Health*. London: Vintage Press.

Daniels, N. and Sabin, J. (2008) *Setting Limits Fairly: Learning to Share Resources for Health*. 2nd edn. New York: Oxford University Press.

Klein, R. and Williams, A. (2000) 'Setting priorities: what is holding us back – inadequate information or inadequate institutions?', in Coulter, A., and Ham, C. (eds) *The Global Challenge of Health Care Rationing*. Buckingham: Open University Press, pp.15–26.

Levi-Faur, D. and Gilad, S. (2004) 'Review: The rise of the British regulatory state – transcending the privatisation debate', *Comparative Politics*, 37(1), pp.105–20.

Longley, D. (1993) *Public Law and Health Service Accountability*. Buckingham: Open University Press.

Majone, G. (1994) 'The rise of the regulatory state in Europe', *West European Politics*, 17(3), pp.77–101.

Majone, G. (1999) 'The regulatory state and its legitimacy problems', *West European Politics*, 22(1), pp.1–24.

McPherson, S. and Sunkin, M. (2020), 'The Dobson-Rawlins pact and the National Institute for Health and Care Excellence: impact of political independence on scientific and legal accountability', *The British Journal of Psychiatry*, 216(4), pp.231–34.

Moran, M. (2000) 'From command state to regulatory state', *Public Policy and Administration*, 15(4), pp.1–13.

Moran, M. (2003) *The British Regulatory State: High Modernism and Hyper-Innovation*. Oxford: Oxford University Press.

Newdick, C. (2014) 'From Hippocrates to commodities: three models of NHS governance', *Medical Law Review*, 22(2), pp.162–79.

NICE (2008) *Social Value Judgements: Principles for the Development of NICE Guidance*. 2nd edn. London: NICE.

NICE (2020) *Our Principles: The Principles that Guide the Development of NICE Guidance and Standards*. London: NICE.

Prosser, T. (1982) 'Towards a critical public law', *Journal of Law and Society*, 9(1), 1–19.

Rawlins, M. (2005) 'Pharmacopolitics and deliberative democracy', *Clinical Medicine*, 5(5), pp.471–5.

Rid, A. (2009) 'Justice and procedure: how does "accountability for reasonableness" result in fair limit-setting decisions?', *Journal of Medical Ethics*, 35(1), pp.12–16.

Shapiro, M. (1992) 'The giving reasons requirement', *University of Chicago Legal Forum*, 1992(1), pp.179–220.

Syrett, K. (2002) 'NICE work? Rationing, review and the "legitimacy problem" in the new NHS', *Medical Law Review*, 10(1), pp.1–27.

Syrett, K. (2004) 'Impotence or importance? Judicial review in an era of explicit NHS rationing' *Modern Law Review*, 67(2), pp.289–304.

Syrett, K. (2007) *Law, Legitimacy and the Rationing of Health Care: A Contextual and Comparative Perspective*. Cambridge: Cambridge University Press.

Syrett, K. (2008) 'NICE and judicial review: enforcing "accountability for reasonableness" through the courts?', *Medical Law Review*, 16(1), pp.127–40.

Syrett, K. (2011) 'Health technology appraisal and the courts: accountability for reasonableness and the judicial model of procedural justice', *Health Economics, Policy and Law*, 6(4), pp. 469–88.

Wang, D. (2017) 'From *Wednesbury* unreasonableness to accountability for reasonableness', *Cambridge Law Journal*, 76(3), pp.642–70.

10 Enhancing the value of public spending on health technology around the world

Ryan Jonathan Sitanggang, Kinanti Khansa Chavarina, Kalipso Chalkidou, Fiona Pearce and Yot Teerawattananon

HTA for universal health coverage

The adoption of the 2030 Sustainable Development Goals in 2015 has led to a commitment from United Nations member states to achieve universal health coverage (UHC), and many have established new, large-scale health insurance schemes to achieve this goal (World Health Organization, 2022). This, however, has undoubtedly put financial pressure on countries to provide health services to the public.

Without a clear, rational process for defining and updating what should be covered in terms of health services and technologies, thousands of discrete, implicit and unpredictable *rationing decisions* will take place between the patient, the service provider and the payer (Center for Global Development, n.d.; Glassman et al., 2016). These decisions are unlikely to result in either an efficient or equitable distribution of health services and resources.

Various methods have been established in different countries to prioritise coverage of health interventions within their health systems (Wiseman et al., 2016). Health technology assessment (HTA), which determines the value of new health technologies compared to existing alternatives, is one such method used to inform the introduction and diffusion of health technologies in the health system. HTA experience and expertise were present at the time of NICE's establishment, as well as in most countries in Western Europe, North America, Australia and New Zealand, although there are differences in criteria, methods and assessment processes. This was not the case in most countries in Asia, Africa and Latin America.

While countries may not require HTA to inform decision-making immediately at the time of UHC introduction, the increasing absolute and relative expenditure on health by governments can fuel interest in using HTA to ensure the additional resources are invested efficiently and equitably. As such, countries in Asia, Africa and Latin America have been increasingly setting up prioritisation processes to inform allocation decisions to support their UHC policies.

DOI: 10.4324/9781003501268-10

The process of establishing an HTA system is recognised as being challenging and complex. However, countries that are yet to implement HTA processes are in a fortunate position to learn from the experiences of countries with mature HTA systems and adopt their best practices. As one of the well-established HTA institutions globally, it is interesting to discover what countries think of NICE. Specifically, what are their perspectives toward NICE's HTA processes and other work? How do these countries learn from NICE?

This chapter explores the international perspective of NICE using findings from a global survey of HTA organisations. It starts with an analysis of NICE's relevance to other HTA organisations, followed by its influence and impact on the processes and methods these HTA organisations have implemented. It also discusses the establishment of NICE International to provide support, technical exchange and assistance to jurisdictions worldwide as they are developing and improving their HTA systems and building local technical capabilities. Finally, the need for HTA support on a global scale and the role of NICE and other HTA agencies are described.

The relevance of NICE to other HTA organisations

A common objective among many jurisdictions is to attain UHC within the context of their respective health systems by building up six critical components that have been defined by the World Health Organization: health service delivery, health workforce, information systems, access to essential medicines, health systems financing, and leadership and governance (World Health Organization, 2010). Of these components, health systems financing is crucial to achieve sustainable UHC. Technical advice and strategic support to maximise health gains within limited healthcare budgets have been increasingly demanded by foreign governments to strengthen their health systems and processes to inform health policy (Chalkidou et al., 2010; Tantivess et al., 2017). The practical approach used by NICE to translate evidence into policy has resulted in better-informed decisions about prioritising investments in health technologies. Such an approach has subsequently been adapted by many jurisdictions to inform their respective healthcare decisions (Tantivess et al., 2017). By evaluating new health technologies through the HTA process, decision-makers can make evidence-informed choices about which interventions to fund and can help healthcare systems distribute limited resources efficiently. This ensures that patients receive healthcare services that are both high in quality and cost-effective.

To assess the international perspective of NICE for the purposes of this chapter, a survey was conducted, and responses were gathered from 14 HTA organisations across Africa, Asia, Australia and Europe (see Table 10.1) that are responsible for producing HTA reports, clinical practice guidelines, and synthesising research evidence to support decision-making in healthcare. Some of

Table 10.1 Responding HTA organisations, jurisdictions where they are based, and the year of establishment

Organisation	Jurisdiction	Year of establishment
Agency for Care Effectiveness	Singapore	2015
Medical Center Hospital of the President's Affairs Administration of the Republic of Kazakhstan	Kazakhstan	2015
Center for Medical and Health Technology Assessment, Department of Pharmaceutical Care, Faculty of Pharmacy, Chiang Mai University	Thailand	2019
Center for Drug Evaluation	Taiwan	2007
China National Health Development Research Center	China	2008
Fondazione Policlinico Universitario Agostino Gemelli IRCCS	Italy	2015
Health Intervention and Technology Assessment Program	Thailand	2007
Instance Nationale de l'Evaluation et de l'Accréditation en Santé	Tunisia	2010
Jawaharlal Institute of Postgraduate Medical Education & Research	India	2020
Mahidol-Oxford Tropical Medicine Research Unit	Thailand	1979
Malaysian Health Technology and Assessment Section	Malaysia	1995
Ministry of Health and Welfare	Taiwan	2007
Royal Australasian College of Surgeons	Australia	1998
Undisclosed*	Bhutan	undisclosed

*the respondent did not disclose the organisation

the organisations solely work on HTA, while some of them also work on other research areas. The organisations serve a variety of sectors, including industry, academia, government and the general public, with the ultimate goal of maximising public health outcomes through a balanced consideration of risks and benefits.

Results from the survey indicated that there is a convergence of vision between NICE and other HTA organisations (see Figures 10.1 and 10.2). One common aim shared by all HTA organisations is the provision of methodologically robust, high-quality HTA to ensure public safety and increased patient access to safe, effective and innovative treatments. This shared goal reflects recognition of the importance of evidence-based decision-making. Similarly, they all shared a commitment to developing and revising clinical practice guidelines to ensure that local clinical practice remains relevant and in line with medical advancements and best practices.

Additionally, the survey results demonstrated that all HTA organisations recognise the importance of forming key strategic partnerships with relevant stakeholders to drive the implementation of their guidance and achieve desired outcomes. Such partnerships are necessary to effectively disseminate clinical or funding recommendations and facilitate their adoption, ensuring that patients receive the highest quality care possible.

Furthermore, the survey highlighted the vision that HTA organisations share of being scientific leaders, driving the research agenda, and developing innovative and data-driven methods to enhance the quality and efficiency of HTA evaluations. By doing so, they can continually evolve and improve their processes and methodologies to better address the needs of patients and other stakeholders.

While some of the similarities between NICE and other mature HTA organisations may be due to the fact that they were established at a similar time, nevertheless, the survey results demonstrated that most HTA organisations, irrespective of their year of establishment, have a shared purpose in their pursuit of better healthcare outcomes for their local populations, which positions NICE as a potential role model for less mature HTA agencies.

Becoming an HTA role model

Role models do not have to be a pioneer, but they should have an impact on an individual's accomplishments, motivation and aspirations by serving as exemplars of behaviour, embodying the achievable and/or providing motivation (Morgenroth et al., 2015). They also demonstrate the type of success one can attain, frequently displaying the necessary attributes to achieve such success and can strengthen an individual's existing goals and drive the adoption of new aspirations (Mcintyre et al., 2011).

For HTA organisations, the function of a role model is not limited to driving vicarious learning or helping to achieve an already desirable goal. Rather, role models can motivate the aspiring organisation to strive towards something novel or superior to their previous pursuits (Morgenroth et al., 2015). The survey respondents perceived that NICE demonstrates behaviours and some of the principles required for success in HTA and sets an achievable example for HTA organisations to aspire to in their efforts to improve healthcare outcomes. They are encouraged by NICE's focus on delivering excellence for patients through innovative thinking and evidence-based decision-making (Charlton et al., 2022; NICE, 2022b). Additionally, NICE's commitment to establishing rigorous standards inspires other HTA organisations to work towards similar objectives (Drummond and Sorenson, 2009).

Be scientific leaders, driving the research agenda and developing innovative and data-driven methods. Use real-world data to resolve issues of uncertainty and improve access to new innovations for patients.   11

Drive the implementation of our guidance, forming key strategic partnerships to make sure it is used. Make sure it delivers improvements and contributes to reducing inequalities, with measures to routinely track adoption.   10

Provide dynamic, living guideline recommendations that are useful, useable, and rapidly updated. Incorporate the latest evidence and newly recommended technologies to maximise uptake and access for patients.   8

Be at the forefront of anticipating and rapidly evaluating new and existing technologies to provide independent, world-leading assessments of value for the system and improved access for patients.   8

Transform our organisation to make sure we have the infrastructure, skills, and capacity to deliver our strategy. Leverage the use of technology to maximise our efficiency and impact.   6

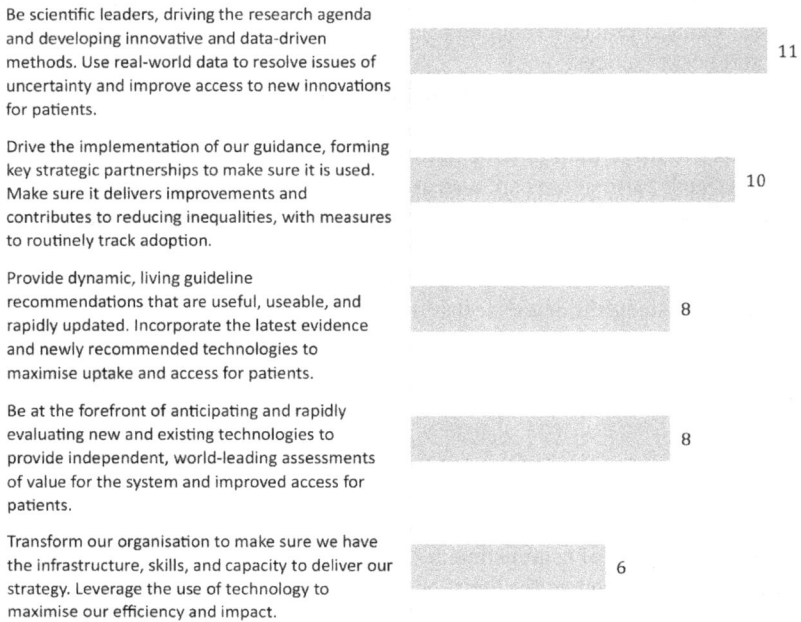

Figure 10.1 Number of HTA organisations with visions aligned with NICE (n=14)

In the previous section, similarities were perceived by the survey respondents between NICE and themselves in terms of vision, technical methodology and fundamental principles. It was interesting to note that these similarities might have encouraged other HTA organisations to emulate NICE's standards and establish their goals accordingly (Mcintyre et al., 2011). The survey revealed that the top three reasons why HTA organisations align their processes and methods with NICE are: 1) the availability of freely accessible products and reports on NICE's activities in English, which are particularly useful in jurisdictions where the capacity to conduct their own HTA is limited; 2) the perception that NICE has a relatively high level of success in the UK; and 3) NICE's good reputation among relevant stakeholders in each of the HTA organisations' jurisdictions.

Some limitations and drawbacks of NICE's processes were also noted by the survey respondents. Specifically, they identified a need for NICE to improve its efforts to reduce health inequalities. Respondents acknowledged that significant progress had been made in this area by NICE through different approaches, such

Use evidence that is relevant, reliable and robust   14

Publish and disseminate recommendations and provide support to encourage their adoption   11

Base recommendations on an assessment of population benefits and value for money   10

Aim to reduce health inequalities   8

Support innovation in the provision and organisation of health and social care services   8

Take into account the advice and experience of people using services and their carers or advocates, health and social care professionals, commissioners, providers and the public   8

Assess the need to update recommendations in line with new evidence   7

Propose new research questions and data collection to resolve uncertainties in the evidence   7

Consider whether it is appropriate to make different recommendations for different groups of people   7

Use independent advisory committees to develop recommendations   6

Describe the approach in process and methods manuals and review them regularly   6

Prepare guidance and standards on topics that reflect national priorities for health and care   6

Offer people interested in the topic the opportunity to comment on and influence recommendations   5

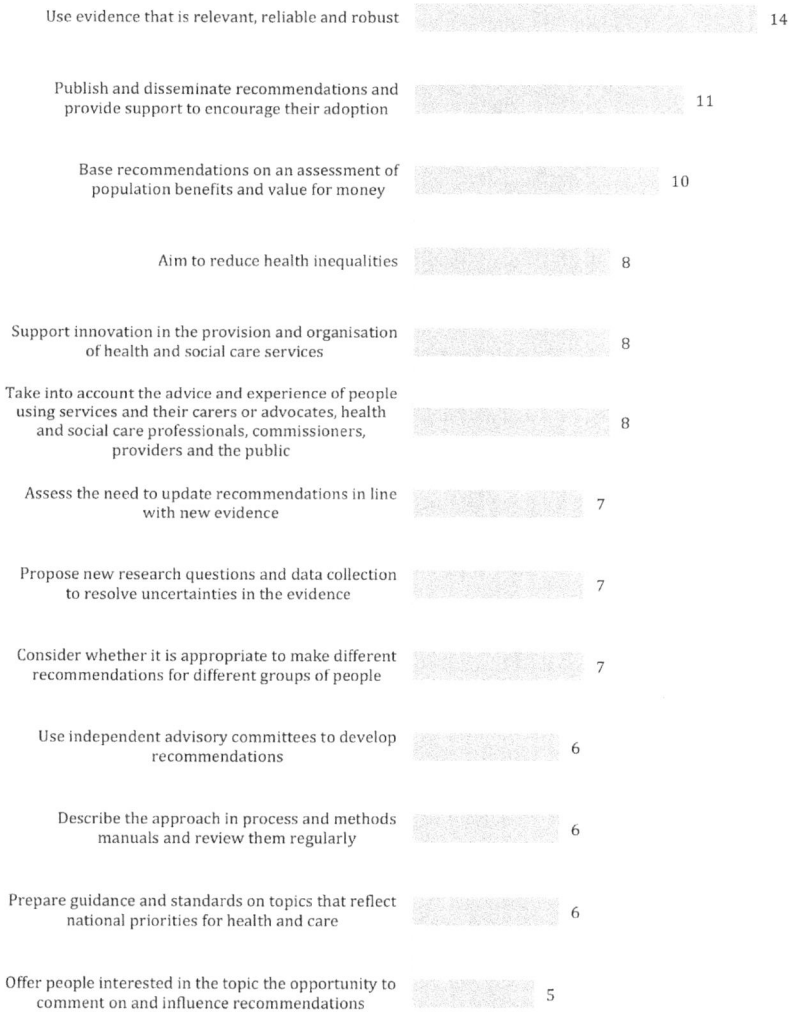

Figure 10.2 Number of HTA organisations with visions aligned with NICE (n=14)

as incorporating feedback from patient groups and recognising potential influences on socio-economic status to different patients while making recommendations. However, despite these efforts, NICE's decisions were still considered to be influenced by political and public opinions, creating additional obstacles to reducing health inequalities. Respondents also suggested that NICE should do more to identify research questions and collect data to address uncertainties in the evidence. Despite these perceived limitations, NICE was still held in high regard by all respondents and was recognised as a role model in the HTA field, particularly for its commitment to ensuring that funding decisions are based on the best available, high-quality evidence.

From role model to making an impact

NICE's success and high-quality products were considered not only to have motivated other HTA organisations to adopt similar processes, but also to have supported decision-making in each jurisdiction. According to respondents, NICE guidelines and technical reports are relatively more detailed and practical compared to their own, and they are routinely retrieved as part of the literature review process to update information on the interventions of interest and provide an additional source of reliable evidence, adapted to the local context as needed, especially in cases where information is not available locally.

Since 2013, some HTA agencies, including NICE, have been using reference cases (endorsed by the International Decision Support Initiative (iDSI) (Wilkinson et al., 2016)) which provide a practical approach to ensuring consistency in technical methods employed and give stakeholders more certainty of the rigour behind the recommendations for resource allocation. The reference case is seen as a cornerstone of NICE's HTA process, making it easier to evaluate different health technologies in a consistent manner and facilitate decision-making across different indications. When conducting analyses, NICE requires companies and independent assessment groups to adhere to a strict set of methods to meet the reference case principles (Wilkinson et al., 2016). Reference cases have also helped researchers embed and reflect a particular population's values on the studied technologies. Most respondents confirmed that they have implemented a reference case that represents the value judgments in their local jurisdictions and considered that it has helped to embed a systematic process of deliberation for their HTA evaluations. In addition to HTA, some jurisdictions, such as Malaysia, also refer to NICE's clinical guidelines to inform healthcare decision-making, which highlights the widespread influence and recognition of NICE as a credible source, not just in HTA but also in clinical practice. Respondents also confirmed that NICE's resources have a significant impact in low- and middle-income countries (LMICs) that have resource limitations and are unable to conduct HTA or develop guidelines locally.

There have been discussions of the issues around NICE's recommendations, such as the questionable provenance of the decision rules (to determine whether or not a technology should be adopted) and the use of limited evidence to assess the clinical benefits of innovative products (Charlton, 2020; Charlton et al., 2022) (see Chapter 5). Yet, despite perceived limitations, five respondents from Australia, Taiwan, Kazakhstan, Malaysia and India considered that NICE's decisions profoundly influenced resource allocation decisions made by policy-makers in their jurisdictions. Unfortunately, specific examples of the type of recommendations that have influenced decision-making were not obtained. But this highlights the crucial role NICE plays in shaping the HTA landscape and decision-making processes in the surveyed jurisdictions.

An example of NICE's influence can be seen during the establishment of the Health Intervention and Technology Assessment Program (HITAP) in Thailand 15 years ago. At that time, less mature HTA agencies lacked support from established HTA agencies. While international collaborations like Health Technology Assessment International (HTAi) and the International Society for Pharmacoeconomics and Outcomes Research (ISPOR) aimed to provide training to enhance technical HTA capacity, they did not address governance issues, implementation processes, or how to drive political support, which are crucial to ensure the long-term success of the HTA agency. To fill this gap, HITAP turned to published information about other HTA agencies' approaches, including NICE, and adapted NICE's approaches in five areas.

The first area was to ensure the quality and comparability of HTA results, with the aim of achieving allocative efficiency, by developing methodological guidelines and a reference case for the Thailand context, similar to NICE's guidelines. In addition, it was mandated that all economic evaluations comply with these standards before they were considered by the Thai government. HITAP also provides annual training and workshops for local researchers and stakeholders to help them conduct HTA studies and interpret the results in line with the reference case.

The second area was using a cost-effectiveness threshold (CET) to determine the value of health technologies. HITAP was the first HTA agency outside of the UK to use an explicit CET, changing it three times over a 15-year period. The first CET in Thailand was THB 100,0000 (GBP 1,780[1]) per QALY in 2008, which was subsequently increased to THB 120,000 (GBP 2,520[2]) per QALY in 2010 and THB 160,000 (GBP 3,040[3]) per QALY in 2013. Currently, HITAP is assessing the impact of changing the CET on drug prices, the probability of drugs being cost-effective and/or included in the benefits package.

The third area was establishing a transparent and participatory HTA process. In the topic nomination process to inform selection for the Universal Coverage Benefit Package, HITAP invites a range of stakeholders, including policy-makers, health professionals, academics, patient associations, civic society and lay citizens. Each group nominates topics which are submitted to a panel

1 THB 1 = GBP 0.018 (2008)
2 THB 1 = GBP 0.021 (2010)
3 THB 1 = GBP 0.019 (2013)

committee comprising representatives of each stakeholder (Lertpitakpong et al., 2008). HITAP and the International Health Policy Program (IHPP), Thailand's research program on national health priorities, assist the panel committee to prioritise topics by using an explicit scoring approach with well-defined parameters and thresholds (Lertpitakpong et al., 2008). The topics nominated are ranked in order and adjusted throughout the deliberation process (Lertpitakpong et al., 2008). Furthermore, reports on whether interventions are included or excluded are publicly accessible (Khampang et al., 2019). Two consultation meetings comprising academics, healthcare providers, healthcare professionals, policy-makers, civic society and lay citizens are held during the start and towards the end of each HTA study (Khampang et al., 2019; Lertpitakpong et al., 2008; Youngkong et al., 2012). The first meeting aims to get agreement among all relevant stakeholders on the scope, policy, and research questions that will be addressed in the HTA, the methodological approach, data sources, and timeline (Khampang et al., 2019; Lertpitakpong et al., 2008). The second meeting aims to verify and validate preliminary results and fine-tune policy recommendations to ensure their validity, relevance, and implementability (Youngkong et al., 2012).

The fourth area that HITAP learned from NICE was the use of 'hard' legal instruments to institutionalise HTA and apply a 'soft power' approach; the former is not always applicable to LMICs because the strength and effectiveness of the rule of law can vary significantly across countries. NICE's early experience of being legally challenged (see Chapter 9) also helped convince HITAP about the need for a different approach in supporting HTA evidence-informed coverage decisions in Thailand. Rather than using its hard power to decide on intervention coverage, HITAP sees itself as a standard setter for HTA and a producer of evidence to support existing decision-making bodies in deciding which pharmaceutical and non-pharmaceutical interventions should be covered under the public health insurance schemes in Thailand. Although the HTA recommendations become indicative rather than directive in this case, effective design and implementation of the deliberative process throughout the HTA process and successful HTA communication can ensure high compliance and impact of HTA work done by HITAP (Teerawattananon et al., 2022). This approach seems to be relevant to many LMICs.

The last area was establishing an international team within the organisation to support emerging HTA systems in other jurisdictions. HITAP played a pivotal role in the adoption of WHO Resolution 67.23 on health intervention and technology assessment supporting universal health coverage (World Health Organization, 2014). HITAP assisted the Chair of NICE in delivering the proposed resolution at the World Health Assembly in May 2014, which was subsequently approved. The resolution highlighted the need for a coordinated global effort to institutionalise HTA and strengthen capacity in countries around the world. By advocating for this resolution and actively participating in its implementation,

HITAP demonstrated its commitment to advancing the field of HTA and supporting the development of effective and sustainable health systems globally. With financial support from international donors and country partner governments, the work of HITAP International Unit further reinforces this commitment by facilitating collaboration and knowledge sharing, as well as supporting capacity building and institutionalisation to governments and institutions across different regions and contexts with the aim to help to build a more robust and interconnected HTA community, ultimately improving the quality and accessibility of healthcare services for people around the world. In turn, HITAP's International Unit enhances HITAP's domestic reputation and impact through collaboration and innovation in the field of HTA. It also helps HITAP to build and retain high-quality researchers in the organisation.

Singapore's national HTA organisation, the Agency for Care Effectiveness (ACE), has also recognised NICE's expertise and has taken steps to adopt some of its best practices (Pearce et al., 2019). This has been achieved by hiring former technical staff from NICE to work at ACE while it was being established, and appointing senior NICE staff to its International Advisory Panel (IAP) in an effort to keep abreast of NICE's process and method changes over time and support local capacity building and methodological development. Members of the IAP, including NICE staff, have provided expert advice on all of ACE's draft process and methods guides for each of its workstreams which has helped ensure that they are aligned with global standards.

During the first years of ACE's establishment, NICE's appraisal documents were often considered as part of the evidence base to inform local decision-making for specific health technologies. They also served as a form of due diligence to confirm similarities and differences in the economic modelling approaches and assumptions used by both agencies to assess the same health technology. NICE's technical documents from their Decision Support Unit (DSU) have also served as helpful training resources for ACE staff to improve their technical capabilities. Over time, NICE's documents have remained important resources. However, in recent years, as ACE has begun to implement parallel regulatory and HTA assessments for certain health technologies, ACE and NICE evaluations now have similar timelines, so NICE's recommendations and technical documents are not always available for ACE staff or decision-makers to refer to.

In May 2023, the Office of Health Economics (OHE) published a report on how NICE's recommendations impact decisions made by other HTA agencies (Henderson et al., 2023). The study employed a mixed methods approach using data from 12 HTA agencies in Australia, Brazil, Canada, France, Israel, Italy, Japan, Poland, Saudi Arabia, South Korea, Sweden, and the United Arab Emirates. The authors reported that these overseas HTA agencies often review NICE appraisals when evaluating similar health technologies. The methodological approach to the evaluation behind NICE's decisions, and the economic model used, often bear more weight in influencing overseas HTA agencies compared to the decision itself. The report also explored the alignment of other HTA agencies' and NICE's methods and processes, including the adoption of cost-effectiveness thresholds and efforts to enhance the transparency and accountability of HTA processes and decision-makers. Adopting NICE's best practices was driven by the HTA agencies' acknowledgment of NICE's reputation as a pioneer in methodological innovation as well as the easy accessibility of NICE's guidance, which is consistent with our findings. Additionally, the OHE report shared other examples of how the UK exercises its 'soft power' to influence overseas HTA agencies, including the speed in which NICE makes decisions and the influence of UK educational institutions in the evaluation process.

These examples portray NICE's well-established position and highlight its proven track record of evolving its methods to meet the demands of the dynamic healthcare landscape, thus allowing it to serve as a role model for less mature or evolving HTA systems. NICE's processes and products have undoubtedly had a positive impact on a global scale. NICE has built a strong reputation in healthcare decision-making, acting as a reliable and credible source to effectively support HTA system development needs and healthcare policy. However, we believe that targeted, direct assistance tailored to the specific needs and circumstances of an HTA organisation could create a more immediate, context-specific impact. Therefore, while NICE's contributions to the international HTA field have been significant through its indirect support, how much impact has NICE made through direct support, especially in LMICs?

Going global: from NICE International to the International Decision Support Initiative

It became apparent very early on in the development of NICE that its approach was generating considerable interest outside the UK. It started with informal invitations to visit other countries and gradually, more formal structures were introduced, e.g., regular meetings with the French (Haute Autorité de Santé – The National Authority for Health) and German (IQWIG [Institut für Qualität und Wirtschaftlichkeit im Gesundheitswesen] – Institute for Quality and Efficiency in Health Care) equivalent organisations. Further developments would benefit from a more coordinated approach. From its inception, NICE formed close links with the Commonwealth Fund, based in the USA, which has an international reputation for health system evaluations, publishing global comparisons of quality (Schneider et al., 2021).

In 2005, the Clinical and Public Health Director was invited to a Commonwealth Fund's Congressional Seminar in Capitol Hill, Washington, in order to present the Institute's early experiences to American policymakers. A year later, he was invited to the Commonwealth Fund Annual Conference. Here, political heads of health systems from around the world meet in Washington to discuss innovation and quality. In 2007, the Associate Director of R&D at NICE was awarded a Harkness Fellowship, and her experiences working in the United States inspired her to consider the international opportunities for NICE. During a visit to Tokyo, Japan, at the launch of the newly established MSc in Health Economics at Keio University, the idea was formulated of creating a designated team to support international efforts to embed HTA in health systems. In 2008, NICE established a dedicated international unit, NICE International, with the aim of supporting HTA capacity building and helping foreign governments make informed decisions on resource allocation. NICE recognised that there was no single approach to help all countries realise this goal. Therefore, it developed a personalised approach to sharing its extensive experience and expertise with other countries while working with local authorities and partners to support methodological development in HTA and strengthen local capabilities.

Since its inception, NICE International has provided advice to over 60 governments on prioritisation decisions. Examples of extensive engagement include Latin American countries, such as Brazil, Colombia, Uruguay and Chile (NICE, n.d.; Pinilla-Dominguez, 2020). NICE International conducted a series of advisory sessions with government agencies and officials to offer advice and support for specific areas of development that were relevant to these four countries (NICE, n.d.). For instance, the sessions in Brazil focused on managed access agreements, analysis and synthesis of qualitative evidence and stakeholder involvement in guidance development (NICE, n.d.). Meanwhile, in Colombia, the focus was on helping establish a national HTA agency as well as developing an EQ-5D-5L valuation set (NICE, n.d.). In Uruguay, the sessions covered the principles of HTA, how to resource an appraisal program and the topic selection process working with their counterpart institutions (NICE, n.d.). The sessions in Chile centered around clinical guideline dissemination and implementation strategies (NICE, n.d.).

The support for these four countries has resulted in several achievements. In Brazil, the HTA unit has undergone substantial modifications, such as the adoption of a multiple-committee structure that comprises separate committees for reviewing pharmaceuticals, non-pharmaceutical technologies, and generating clinical guidelines (NICE, 2022b). Furthermore, these committees' memberships have been broadened to include medical doctors and methodologists from hospital based HTA units. Moreover, lay members can now attend meetings. The unit recently held a public consultation to solicit feedback on the possibility of including a cost-effectiveness threshold in its work.

In Colombia, the National Agency for HTA (Instituto de Evaluación Tecnológica en Salud – IETS) has taken significant steps to promote public participation in the HTA processes (NICE, n.d.). IETS has developed a manual for patient involvement and implemented engagement strategies to encourage the public to share their opinions and insights on the health technology (NICE, n.d.). As a result of these efforts, HTA processes in Colombia have become more inclusive and transparent.

Uruguay has achieved notable progress by creating a unit within the Ministry of Health (MOH), namely the Health Assessment Division (HAD-MoH) for HTA, comprising professionals trained in HTA. The agency has laid out its preliminary organisational framework and methods for evaluating health technologies and is now beginning to put them into practice upon receiving requests from the national healthcare system (NICE, n.d.).

In Chile, the Department of HTA and Evidence-Based Health has refined its implementation support offer and incorporated learnings into its strategy and tools (NICE, n.d.). Furthermore, Chile is considering the creation of an independent HTA agency. The relationship between Chile and the UK has been strengthened, and the UK has become an important reference for Chile in relation to HTA.

In Asia, NICE International helped Vietnam's Ministry of Health to adapt international evidence on stroke management to the local setting and identified simple and effective measures to improve the quality of stroke management. The quality standards developed through this process are currently being implemented in major public hospitals in Hanoi. In one of India's states, Kerala, NICE International helped to reduce the maternal mortality rate from 88 to 66 per 100,000 live births at that time (Maya, 2014; Rajagopal, 2013; Tantivess et al., 2017). This was done by adapting NICE's evidence-informed guidelines into locally applicable and quantifiable performance metrics, contextualized through a transparent and collaborative process (Tantivess et al., 2017). The programme encompassed training for all labour personnel, the rollout of a new maternity register, as well as purchasing and distributing new disposable delivery kits (Tantivess et al., 2017).

In 2015, a triennial review of NICE commissioned by the UK government recommended that NICE should explore opportunities to expand the services of NICE International and NICE Scientific Advice and consider alternative models or sectors for delivery. This was in the context of a range of NHS initiatives seeking to influence health care in other countries. In its report, *Strengthening Health Systems in Developing Countries* (UK Parliament, 2014), the International Development Committee specifically mentioned NICE International:

Demand for NHS staff does not end with doctors and nurses. Though often criticised at home, the NHS is held in high international regard and many countries would greatly benefit from the assistance of those expert in managing and financing such a successful health system. In turn, NHS managers would benefit from tackling familiar problems in unfamiliar settings. This is a challenge to traditional development models and DFID [Department for International Development] must be sufficiently agile to adapt to changing and increasingly complex needs. NICE International is a successful example of how NHS expertise can benefit overseas systems, and leverage funds from other donors in the process. **We recommend that DFID establish a clear strategy for how UK government should work in partnership with the NHS to support overseas health systems**.

An Institute internal review of how to respond to this request resulted in a proposal that the Scientific Advice team, which provided advice to the pharmaceutical industry on how best to optimise its submissions on new drugs to the Institute, should remain as part of the structure, but the team managing NICE International was to be encouraged to find alternative structures and sources of funding.

During the following year, a range of options was discussed with little consensus on the best way to achieve global influence. The main tension was between those advocating a commercially viable consulting agency model or continuing the academic collaborative nonprofit support model. In 2016, after a year of discussions, the staff constituting NICE International moved to Imperial College London and continued its work under the auspices of the International Decision Support Initiative (iDSI). The NICE International brand remained with NICE. In 2022 it published its three-year strategy articulating two main aims: 1) improving healthcare outcomes across the world by sharing the learning and expertise of NICE internationally, enhancing NICE's reputation as a world-leading institution; and 2) establishing international collaborative relationships aligned with NICE's priority areas (NICE, 2023).

This suggests a less ambitious programme than originally envisaged, with less emphasis on development, institutional partnerships and providing public information on its work with LMICs. The strategy is clear that, in order to deliver the service offering sustainably, NICE International will be required to operate on a not-for-profit, cost-recovery basis. This is in line with the Regulations governing NICE's constitution and functions (2013), which allow for operating on a commercial basis. NICE International will aim to recover the cost of its advisory role when working with international organisations and sharing NICE's learnings and expertise under strategic ambition.

iDSI continues its international activities and networking, networking, recruiting new partners, e.g., The London School of Hygiene and Tropical Medicine, University of Strathclyde, the UK-based Center for Global Development, the Norwegian Institute of Public Health, Institute for Clinical Effectiveness and Health Policy, Radboud University Medical Center, China National Health Development and Research Center, Africa Central Disease Control, Kenya Medical Research Institute, Wellcome Trust and Clinton Health Access Initiative. iDSI operates through funding from the Bill & Melinda Gates Foundation, The Rockefeller Foundation and the UK Foreign, Commonwealth and Development Office. At the time of writing, the funding of iDSI, mostly reliant on Gates, is under threat. If not renewed, the iDSI partnership will have concluded a ten-year journey, starting with NICE International, and dedicated to building partnerships and promoting the use of evidence and deliberative processes in decision-making around the world.

This chapter has described NICE's global influence and highlights, like much of the Institute's activities, how it has evolved and changed over the years. Whilst the current NICE International page on the Institute's website documents case studies on engagement activities, it has limited material predating 2019, including the wealth of the NICE International work and related partnerships. For ease of access, all of NICE International's annual reports spanning 2009 to 2015 (NICE, 2009–2015) and work referred to by the UK Parliament (NICE, 2023; The UK Parliament, 2014), which laid the foundation for the later international engagement activities that NICE now concentrates on, can be accessed online at https://www.hitap.net/en/187711.

Looking forward

Apart from supporting other agencies in conducting and using HTA to inform policy, NICE has leveraged international networks to advance its own work. Through its partnerships with other HTA organisations (which currently stands at eight organisations at the time of writing), comprising the Canadian Agency for Drugs and Technologies in Health, Healthcare Improvement Scotland (Scottish Medicines Consortium and Scottish Health Technologies Group), Health Technology Wales, All Wales Therapeutics & Toxicology Centre, the Australian Government's Department of Health and Aged Care, Institut national d'excellence en santé et services sociaux (Quebec) and Pharmac (New Zealand), NICE is promoting collaboration, sharing expertise, and addressing common challenges (NICE, 2022a). NICE has also taken an approach to advancing the field of HTA through education and training initiatives with the London School of Economics with a formation of a formal international programme on HTA (London School of Economics and Political Science, n.d.).

Looking ahead, it is evident that LMICs, as well as donor agencies financed by wealthy country donations, increasingly recognise the importance of UHC and HTA; especially after the pandemic, which has underscored the interdependence of public health, national security, and economic development. With the advancement of new health technologies entering the market, the need for governments to carefully justify funding decisions will become more pressing as they balance the benefits and costs of each technology, among other considerations. It is also essential to ensure that these technologies are accessible and affordable to everyone, regardless of their economic status. This will require collaboration between governments, the private sector and civil society.

In this context, the role of HTA agencies will be vital to support governments in making resource allocation decisions. It is believed that NICE and other successful HTA agencies could play a significant role in facilitating the development of new HTA agencies in the future. As the HTA community continues to grow, NICE's position as a point of reference is likely to remain. However, knowledge sharing between countries and public service institutions is better viewed as a global public good than a money-making exercise. Perhaps now is an opportunity for the UK government to commit to financing NICE International and revert to the original model of peer-to-peer support, at arm's length from commercial or healthcare industry engagements and with a clear public good intention. As Southern HTA institutions become well established and to the extent, they stay true to their non-profit character, it is believed that South–South partnerships are set to grow stronger and more impactful than during the early days of NICE International. This can only be a good thing which all those involved in the establishment of global support for HTA development, including NICE International, HITAP's International Unit, and iDSI, could only have dreamed of!

References

Center for Global Development. (n.d.) 'Priority-setting in health: building institutions for smarter public spending'. Available at: https://www.cgdev.org/media/priority-setting-health-building-institutions-smarter-public-spending (Accessed: 15 February 2023).

Chalkidou, K., Levine, R. and Dillon, A. (2010) 'Helping poorer countries make locally informed health decisions', *British Medical Journal,* 341:c3651.

Charlton, V. (2020) 'NICE and fair? Health technology assessment policy under the UK's National Institute for Health and Care Excellence, 1999–2018', *Health Care Analysis,* 28, pp.193–227.

Charlton, V., Lomas, J. and Mitchell, P. (2022) 'NICE's new methods: putting innovation first, but at what cost?', *British Medical Journal,* 379:e071974.

Drummond, M. and Sorenson, C. (2009) 'Nasty or nice? A perspective on the use of health technology assessment in the United Kingdom', *Value in Health,* 12 Suppl 2, pp.S8–13.

Glassman, A., Giedion, U., Sakuma, Y. and Smith, P. C. (2016). 'Defining a health benefits package: what are the necessary processes?', *Health Systems and Reform,* 2, pp.39–50.

Henderson, N., Brassel, S., O'Neill, P., Allen, R., Largeron, N. and Garau, M. (2023) *Do NICE's Decision Outcomes Impact International HTA Decision-making?,* OHE Contract Research Report. London: Office of Health Economics. Available from: https://www.ohe.org/?post_type=publications&p=5628&preview=true (Accessed 18 February 2023).

Khampang, R., Khuntha, S., Hadnorntun, P., Kumluang, S., Anothaisintawee, T., Tanuchit, S., Tantivess, S. and Teerawattananon, Y. (2019) 'Selecting topic areas for developing quality standards in a resource-limited setting', *British Medical Journal Open Quality,* 8:e000491.

Lertpitakpong, C., Chaikledkaew, U., Thavornchatoensap, M., Tantivess, S., Praditsitthikorn, N., Youngkong, S., Yothasamut, J., Udomsuk, K., Sinthitichai, K. and Teerawattananon, Y. (2008) 'A determination of topics for health technology assessment in Thailand: making decision makers involved', *Journal of the Medical Association of Thailand,* 91, pp.S100–9.

London School of Economics and Political Science. (n.d.) 'Executive MSc healthcare decision-making, in collaboration with NICE'. Available at https://www.lse.ac.uk/ study-at-lse/Graduate/degree-programmes-2023/Executive-MSc-Healthcare-Deci sion-Making (Accesssed 28 September 2023).

Maya, C. (2014) 'Kerala's MMR comes down to 66', *The Hindu* (5 January). Available at: https://www.thehindu.com/news/national/kerala/keralas-mmr-comes-down-to-66/ article5541348.ece (Accessed 18 February 2023).

Mcintyre, R.B., Paulson, R.M., Taylor, C.A., Morin, A.L. and Lord, C.G. (2011) 'Effects of role model deservingness on overcoming performance deficits induced by stereo-type threat', *European Journal of Social Psychology*, 41, pp.301–11.

Morgenroth, T., Ryan, M.K. and Peters, K. (2015) 'The motivational theory of role mod-eling: how role models influence role aspirants' goals', *Review of General Psychology*, 19, **pp.**465–83.

NICE (n.d.) 'Health technology assessment in Latin America – advancing together'. Available at: https://case-studies.nice.org.uk/LatinAmerica/index.html (Accessed 30 March 2023).

NICE (2009–2015) 'NICE International Review' Available at: https://www.hitap.net/ en/187711 (Accessed 2 October 2023).

NICE (2022a) 'NICE partners with international health technology assessment bodies to boost collaboration on shared opportunities and challenges'. Available. at: https:// www.nice.org.uk/news/article/nice-partners-with-international-health-technology-assessment-bodies. (Accessed 15 February 2023).

NICE (2022b) 'NICE publishes new combined methods and processes manual and topic selection manual for its health technology evaluation programmes'. Available at: https://www.nice.org.uk/news/article/nice-publishes-new-combined-methods-and-processes-manual-and-topic-selection-manual-for-its-health-technology-evaluation-programmes (Accessed 15 February 2023).

NICE (2023) 'About NICE International'. Available at: https://www.nice.org.uk/about/ what-we-do/nice-international/about-nice-international (Accessed 30 March 2023).

Pearce, F., Lin, L., Teo, E., Ng, K. and Khoo, D. (2019) 'Health technology assess-ment and its use in drug policies: Singapore', *Value in Health Regional Issues*, 18, pp.176–85.

Pinilla-Dominguez, P. (2020) 'NICE International representatives complete working visit to Latin America'. Available at: https://www.nice.org.uk/news/blog/nice-interna tional-representatives-complete-working-visit-to-latin-america (Accessed 18 February 2023).

Rajagopal, K. (2013) 'Where grieving mothers struggle to find answers', *The Hindu* (3 May). Available at: https://www.thehindu.com/news/national/kerala/where-griev ing-mothers-struggle-to-find-answers/article4677737.ece (Accessed 18 February 2023).

Schneider, E.C., Shah, A., Doty, M.M., Tikkanen, R., Fields, K. and Williams II, R.D. (2021) *Mirror, Mirror 2021: Reflecting Poorly*. Online. Available at: https://www. commonwealthfund.org/publications/fund-reports/2021/aug/mirror-mirror-2021-re flecting-poorly (Accessed 28 September 2023).

Tantivess, S., Chalkidou, K., Tritasavit, N. and Teerawattananon, Y. (2017) 'Health Tech-nology Assessment capacity development in low- and middle-income countries: expe-riences from the international units of HITAP and NICE', *F1000Research*, 6, 2119.

Teerawattananon, Y., Dabak, S., Culyer, A.J., Mills, A., Kingkaew, P. and Isaranuwatchai, W. (2022) *Fifteen Lessons from Fifteen Years of the Health Intervention and Technol-ogy Assessment Program (HITAP), Thailand*. Unpublished.

UK Parliament (2014) *Strengthening Health Systems in Developing Countries – International Development Committee: Fifth Report*. Available at: https://publications. parliament.uk/pa/cm201415/cmselect/cmintdev/246/24608.htm#a18 (Accessed 30 March 2023).

Wilkinson, T., Sculpher, M.J., Claxton, K., Revill, P., Briggs, A., Cairns, J.A., Teerawat-tananon, Y., Asfaw, E., Lopert, R., Culyer, A.J. and Walker, D.G. (2016) 'The International Decision Support Initiative reference case for economic evaluation: an aid to thought', *Value in Health,* 19, pp.921–28.

Wiseman, V., Mitton, C., Doyle-Waters, M.M., Drake, T., Conteh, L., Newall, A.T., Onwujekwe, O. and Jan, S. (2016) 'Using economic evidence to set healthcare priorities in low-income and lower-middle-income countries: a systematic review of methodological frameworks', *Health Economics,* 25 Suppl 1, pp.140–61.

World Health Organization (2010) *Monitoring the Building Blocks of Health Systems: A Handbook of Indicators and their Measurement Strategies,* Geneva: World Health Organization.

World Health Organization (2014) *Health Intervention and Technology Assessment in Support of Universal Health Coverage.* Geneva: World Health Organization. Available at: https://apps.who.int/iris/handle/10665/162870 (Accessed 15 February 2023).

World Health Organization (2022) *Universal Health Coverage (UHC).* Geneva: World Health Organization. Available at: https://www.who.int/news-room/fact-sheets/detail/universal-health-coverage-(uhc) (Accessed 10 February 2023).

Youngkong, S., Baltussen, R., Tantivess, S., Mohara, A. & Teerawattananon, Y. (2012) 'Multicriteria decision analysis for including health interventions in the universal health coverage benefit package in Thailand', *Value in Health,* 15, pp.961–70.

11 Conclusion

NICE from the past into the future

Peter Littlejohns, David J. Hunter and Keith Syrett

Survival in a changing world

NICE has existed through some of the best and the worst periods in the history of the NHS. During its lifetime, many other NHS institutions concerned with quality and innovation have come and gone, including the Health Protection Agency, the National Treatment Agency for Substance Misuse, Public Health Observatories, the Modernisation Agency, NHS University, NHS Institute for Learning Skills and Innovation, National Patient Safety Agency, the National Clinical Assessment Service and Public Health England – and this list is not exhaustive. So why has NICE survived and, indeed, thrived? It was certainly not a foregone conclusion. In the early days, it was not just the pharmaceutical industry and patient advocacy groups lobbying for the end of NICE. In 2000, the editor of the *British Medical Journal* (BMJ) (Smith, 2000: 1363) wrote:

> Despite the protestations of its boss, the National Institute for Clinical Excellence (NICE) is an instrument for rationing health care. Unfortunately, it's not a very good one. A government with spine would learn from the failings of NICE and move on to version 2. Perhaps this is a job for after the next election, whoever wins.

He continued (ibid.: 1364):

> One failing of NICE is that it's living a double lie. The first lie – which is as Orwellian as its name – is to deny that it's about rationing health care, which might be defined as 'denying effective interventions'. Denying ineffective interventions is not rationing; rather it's what the Americans call a 'no brainer'. The population is smart enough both to know that NICE is rationing health care and that rationing of health care is inevitable. The second, and related, lie is to give the impression that if the evidence supports a treatment then it's made available and if it doesn't it isn't. In other words, the whole messy problem of deciding which interventions to make available can

DOI: 10.4324/9781003501268-11

be decided with some data and a computer. It's a technical problem. This lie corrupts the concept of evidence-based medicine, which the *BMJ* has long championed. The evidence supports decision-making, but the evidence can't make the decision. The values of the patient or the community must be part of the decision.

He concluded (ibid.):

Probably NICE had to exist in order for us to begin to think about something better. A single body cannot 'solve' the problem of rationing, but Britain would benefit from a body that admits it is about rationing, works openly, uses evidence, looks right across health care, incorporates ethical thinking systematically into its judgments, is more distant from politicians and the pharmaceutical industry, and is directly accountable to the public. Let's call it CHOR – the Committee for Honest and Open Rationing.

However four years later he had changed his tune. In another *BMJ* editorial called 'The triumph of NICE' (Smith, 2004), he wrote:

The National Institute for Clinical Excellence (NICE) and the Commission for Health Improvement (CHI) were both introduced in the NHS plan of 1998. Six years on, CHI is dead but NICE is conquering the world. NICE worked but 'nasty' (as CHI was initially known) failed – perhaps because it wasn't nasty enough. NICE may prove to be one of Britain's greatest cultural exports, along with Shakespeare, Newtonian physics, the Beatles, Harry Potter, and the Teletubbies.

Probably the key reason for this change of heart was that NICE addressed his concern that 'the values of the patient or the community must be part of the decision'. This culminated in NICE publishing *Social Value Judgements* in 2005, subsequently updated in 2008 to reflect its expansion into public health (NICE, 2008). This version existed until 2020 when it was replaced with *Our Principles* (NICE, 2020). How these values were interpreted by NICE, introduced into its processes, and the significance of the change to principles, are addressed in several of the preceding chapters (2, 4, 5, and 6).

It is important to note that the thinking of NICE did not stagnate during this 12 year period. Following the standing down of the ethics advisory committee that advised NICE on the 2008 document, the Clinical and Public Health Director together with Albert Weale, Professor of Political Theory and Public Policy, created an informal social values group (consisting of ethicists, political scientists, lawyers, public health practitioners) at University College London and Kings College London. This work culminated in NICE hosting a workshop in 2012 to explore how values were being integrated into deliberation internationally.

A special journal edition described the activities in ten countries and heralded the start of a new international research programme (Littlejohns et al., 2012). The Clinical and Public Health Director left NICE in 2013 to carry this work forward, although contact and collaboration with the Institute was maintained. A second international workshop was held in 2015 with senior members of the Institute in attendance, including the new NICE chairman Professor Sir David Haslam, when public involvement in deliberation was explored across a range of countries (Weale et al., 2016). In 2018, a Rockefeller Residency in Bellagio facilitated the writing up of the project (Littlejohns et al., 2019a). In all, representatives from 14 countries and the World Bank were involved. However this group's views diverged following NICE's shift from values to principles (Littlejohns et al., 2019b).

This example of NICE's responsiveness to evaluation and analysis, both positive and negative, is a common theme throughout its history. It has been adept at adjusting its relationship with key stakeholders through modifying its processes and methods. Most chapters provide examples of how this was achieved. Perhaps the most important is how its appraisal methods evolved, highlighted in Chapter 2. Regarding the acceptability of methods it is informative to compare NICE's experiences with the other new organisation established to support the Blair government's strategy to improve quality in the NHS. The Commission for Health Improvement (CHI) was created in 1999 to assess quality of NHS organisations, including how well they implemented NICE guidance.

Over the subsequent 25 years these two organisations followed very different paths. CHI's initial methodology was based on inspection, with an aim of supporting improvement. Four years after its establishment, CHI was subsumed by the Healthcare Commission, officially the Commission for Healthcare Audit and Inspection (CHAI) (Health and Social Care (Community Health and Standards) Act 2003). At the time it was widely believed that senior management at CHI and the then Secretary of State Alan Milburn disagreed over how CHI should operate. Peter Homa (CHI CEO) favoured a facilitating, enabling approach to quality improvement, while Milburn preferred a more punitive, 'big stick' approach. Using a very different methodology to CHI, with an emphasis on analysis of information, CHAI, under the leadership of Professor Sir Ian Kennedy, was in existence for five years until its responsibilities were taken over by the Care Quality Commission (CQC) in 2009 (Health and Social Care Act (Commencement No. 9, Consequential Amendments and Transitory, Transitional and Saving Provisions) Amendment Order 2009), which applied yet another methodology to its task and returned to an emphasis on inspection. However, in 2013 CQC was very much in the news. A series of national reports were published and television exposés were broadcast, culminating in the Francis Inquiry (Francis, 2012), which highlighted the poor quality of care in certain hospitals and care homes. Coalition health ministers talked about 'a poor culture' and 'acceptance of the mediocre' by many workers in the

NHS. Interestingly, much of the negative publicity concentrated on the NHS approach to monitoring quality and the responsible institution, rather than the failing hospitals themselves. Such was the outcry about the CQC that new senior staff were appointed and yet another change in its approach to inspection with an emphasis on professional leadership was announced in the House of Commons by the Prime Minister (BBC News, 2013).

At the heart of all these changes was a lack of agreement on the methods to be used and the differing cultures of the two organisations (Littlejohns et al., 2017), the latter being especially important, as described in Chapter 3. However, it was perhaps inevitable, given the differing size and complexities of monitoring and improving the quality of every organisation in the NHS, without a consensus on methods, that CHI would be vulnerable to government interventions. Historically, ministers have been only too keen to meddle in those inspection-type bodies focused on NHS delivery (i.e. waiting lists, meeting performance targets etc.), whose work carries a political cost because of its visibility to the public and media. However, NICE's 'rationing' remit has been an area from which (for the most part), ministers are keen to stand back, given its potential as an ethical and political minefield. Even in those exceptional cases where politicians did meddle (e.g. Hewitt over Herceptin, and Cameron over the Cancer Drugs Fund: see Chapter 3), they got their fingers burned. The scientific, evidence-based nature of NICE's methodology and work also made it more 'technical' and less susceptible to Ministerial interference (Syrett, 2003), especially when combined with its organisational independence from government. This may have helped it survive various attempts to cull quangos, as did the strong support and respect from key officials in the Department of Health/Department of Health and Social Care.

It should be noted that the Francis Inquiry also had implications for NICE, but although these caused some difficulties, they were not as dramatic as those for CQC. NICE was invited by NHS England to develop guidance on safe nursing levels. The first guidance on safe nursing levels in acute care was published in July 2014.[1] This was supposed to be the first of a proposed suite of guidance covering all areas of the hospital; however, the commission was rescinded by NHS England. It is likely that the implications of defining specific nursing numbers for all aspects of care were too daunting to be manageable by an NHS under severe financial and staffing levels challenges. In this case the reputation of NICE was not diminished as NHS created a consortium of institutions – the National Quality Board (of which NICE was a part), and NHS Improvement subsequently issued these as 'support documents' rather than guidance.[2]

---

1 See https://www.nice.org.uk/guidance/sg1.
2 See https://www.england.nhs.uk/nursingmidwifery/safer-staffing-nursing-and-midwifery/safe-staffing-improvement-resources-for-specific-settings/

While adapting its methods (always keeping to the key principles of openness, transparency and engagement) was the most visible means of NICE responding to stakeholder concerns, it was not the only way. As discussed in more detail in Chapter 8, a key feature of NICE was the multiplicity of stakeholders with which it interacted, including patients and the public, health professionals and academics, Royal Colleges and NHS organisations, the therapeutics industry, and the Department of Health, not to mention the professional and public press. NICE functioned at the interface of all these stakeholders and needed to understand their priorities and communicate in a way relevant to each. An early priority of the Institute was to never turn down an opportunity to communicate its message. However difficult an interview or presentation was likely to be – and they could be very difficult – the Institute would field a suitable person to present its case at conferences, or on radio and television. The level of independence that NICE enjoyed from government facilitated this, as did the longevity of the senior staff in post being able to display and understand a corporate history often lacking in many other NHS institutions (see Chapter 3). Another feature of maintaining stakeholder trust was the emphasis on partnership and involvement through the creation of the national collaborating centres. The cessation of this mode of working in 2022 means finding new ways of ensuring that the Institute's role in guidance development remains relevant and acceptable, especially as institutions such as Royal Colleges which previously developed guidance will most likely take on this role again.

How has NICE performed?

In sum, key to NICE's survival across 25 years was its capacity to adapt; but it was also assisted by the nature of its work, and its capacity to avoid attracting too much ministerial attention. Over the years, NICE has been seen to undertake a range of roles addressing issues of quality in the health and social care systems within its broad directives, as issued by government.

The roles of NICE in its first 25 years

1. NICE is an instrument of fairness, for example in eliminating post-code prescribing or in providing a voice, via the notion of opportunity costs, for patients who might otherwise be neglected.
2. NICE is an instrument for the more efficient use of resources, either in the specific form (as proposed in Chapter 2) of QALY maximization, or in a vaguer form understood as getting best value for money out of the NHS budget.
3. NICE is an instrument for determining what should be included in the package of health care that the NHS supplies, a role that is performed by a number of different organisations in other health care systems.

4. NICE is intended to be an instrument of depoliticising difficult health care decisions, a role that some (Klein and Maybin, 2012) have suggested could never be successful.
5. NICE is an instrument for disguising the unpalatable truth about rationing (which was Smith's first view: see above).
6. NICE is an instrument for applying modern scientific understanding to the problems associated with priority-setting (which was Smith's second view: see above).
7. NICE is a mechanism to encourage the NHS to innovate and adopt new interventions more quickly.
8. NICE should apply principles of fairness, effectiveness and efficiency to Public Health and Social Care.
9. NICE should seek to reduce use of inappropriate, ineffective or cost-ineffective interventions.

Across the chapters of this book we have seen how some roles have been emphasised more than others during the last 25 years. Any assessment of NICE's performance will need to first decide which of these roles are considered to be the most important. Chapters 2, 5 and 6 suggest that innovation has dominated, to the detriment of fairness, in the assessment of new expensive pharmaceuticals. However, much of this debate depends on whether the main purpose of NICE is considered to be to maximise QALYs.

Wilson argues in Chapter 6 that health quality need not be synonymous with this aspiration. He argues that opportunity costs can be considered in one of two ways. Either opportunity cost is just one of a number of ethically relevant concerns: for example, in the case of funding intensive treatment units, it may be not just ethically *permissible* to pursue a policy that leads to more health being displaced than is created, but arguably ethically *obligatory* to do so. Or, alternatively, a broader vision of what counts as an opportunity cost could be adopted, such that we think of the opportunity costs of particular interventions in terms of the displacement of *value*, rather than *health*. In the latter case, opportunity can be considered to be any aspect of improvement for a health system, rather than presupposing that it is only the maximisation of health that matters.

In contrast, in Chapter 2, Sculpher and colleagues appear to consider QALY maximisation as dominant, and provide suggestions for an immediate remedy for NICE to adopt. However even this proposed solution might prove problematic as it seems to shift normative aspects of decision-making back downstream in ways that would likely (re)introduce inequality and incoherence. NICE seems to have 'done best' when weighing up complex normative considerations through deliberation, not simply by assessing evidence.

Looking ahead: lessons from the past 25 Years

As NICE faces the future, is there learning from its first quarter-century that might be useful to heed? This is not an attempt to predict the future, but to set out what we know to be challenges in need of attention. Some of these are not new but have been overlooked by successive governments. Whatever happens, the NHS will continue to evolve and change; but in what direction will depend upon where government priorities lie, and these will have implications for NICE.

In the aftermath of Covid-19, there is a view that 'active government' (in contrast to the libertarian view that government is best when it governs least) may be making a comeback, especially in light of a possible change of government, and that protecting the public from health threats needs to be given a higher priority (Littlejohns et al., 2024). Having been hollowed out for the past 12 years or so, there is a resurgence of support for investing in and rebuilding the public realm. How far such thinking will determine future government priorities when it comes to health is unclear. But there is at least more attention being given to the widening health gap and how to tackle it. As part of this, health and wealth are seen as inextricably linked – it is not possible to have one without the other. Prior to the pandemic, the focus was on wealth rather than health. But what Covid-19 demonstrated beyond all doubt was the need for a healthy workforce if wealth was to be created and distributed appropriately.

The financial and staffing pressures on the NHS arising not only from Covid-19, but also from over a decade of austerity will take a long time to reverse. In the meantime, there is talk of 'reform' once again, despite the NHS in England being in the midst of major reform arising from the Health and Care Act 2022. For example, the *Times* Health Commission established in January 2023 will produce recommendations for reform in 2024 (Sylvester, 2023). The Labour Party has also included NHS reform as one of its five missions (Labour Party, 2023). What further reform might entail remains unclear. At one extreme, there are those who argue that talk of reform is a dangerous distraction which plays into the right-wing think-tanks which want to replace the NHS though a mix of social insurance and privatisation. The answer, they claim, is to fund the NHS appropriately and put in place a workforce plan to secure staff recruitment and retention. Also, greater attention needs to be given to health prevention and promotion and to resolving the crisis in social care.

At the other extreme are those who want a more radical shake-up of the system; although what would emerge from such an exercise is unclear. The problem with this reform agenda is that in the past the NHS has been subjected to numerous inquiries and all have concluded that there is no better system in terms of funding than the one which exists. Replacing a tax-funded system with a social insurance model would be expensive and disruptive for what its opponents argue would be minimal gain.

Whatever emerges from these various maximal or minimal reform efforts, they will have implications for NICE. Improved funding for the NHS might enable NICE guidance to carry more weight when it comes to investment decisions in new treatments. Also, adopting a whole system approach to health rather than a narrow focus on health care has implications for NICE's role in public health and social care. These sectors merit a higher profile and priority within NICE. Whether it is fit for purpose in this regard is not clear. Certainly the loss of the Centre for Public Health Excellence and the decommissioning of the Social Care Institute for Excellence for producing social care guidance mean that new approaches will have to be developed and tested.

Irrespective of any further structural changes which may emerge in health system policy, there are two areas where change is likely. First is the increasing pace of change which is in part driven by technology but also by developments in media and communications. This raises an issue for NICE, which is committed to in-depth rigour in its evidence-based medicine approach. As noted in several of the preceding chapters (see Chapters 2, 4, 5 and 6), NICE has increasingly moved towards a focus upon innovation, however, the length of time it takes to reach decisions and produce guidance remains problematic. Enabling the production of timely, relevant, high-quality guidance in fast-moving areas of medicine will be a test of NICE's continuing value and relevance.

The focus on science and technology has taken on a greater urgency with a government concerned about the lack of growth in the UK. This is a consequence of several factors, notably 12 years of austerity and falling investment, the impact of Brexit on all aspects of the economy including a shortage of labour, and the aftermath of Covid-19 on the economy, on health inequalities, and the state of population health more generally. A renewed focus on the life sciences and innovation has been set out at some length by two former party leaders, Tony Blair and William Hague, in a joint report (Blair and Hague, 2023). The authors argue that Britain's future depends on a new age of invention and innovation with science and technology at its core. At the heart of these are developments in artificial intelligence, biotech, climate tech and other fields which will have major impacts on our economic and social systems.

As considered in Chapters 5 and 6, where NICE fits into this agenda has been an ongoing concern for many years, although it may be becoming more acute given the renewed political interest in the life sciences and related areas. Certainly, for a time NICE was seen as part of the problem rather than the solution. A review of UK health research funding commissioned by the government found that there was a need for a more systematic approach to the adoption of new technologies and interventions in the NHS (Cooksey, 2006) and that, in particular, the government should consider ways of bringing drugs that address UK health priorities to market faster, since the UK 'is at risk of failing to reap the full economic, health and social benefits that [its] public investment in health research should generate' (ibid.: para. 6). To achieve this, Cooksey proposed that

NICE be involved earlier in the process of development to accelerate assessment of clinical and cost-effectiveness and that it should work with the pharmaceutical industry to identify new medicines under development that might be suited to piloting earlier NICE involvement. In response, NICE commissioned Sir Ian Kennedy to consider the value of innovation and other benefits (Kennedy, 2009). The detailed study produced 25 recommendations, the majority of which took their cue from the Cooksey report's recommendations and endorsed many of them. These included that NICE 'should be more active in explaining its role and decisions and develop a strategy to achieve this' (ibid.: 19); 'should work closely with Pharma in a number of areas, such as formulating a definition of innovation through which Pharma can signal as early as possible that a product may constitute an innovation as defined, and ensuring that the data required by NICE to make this judgement is generated' (ibid.: 20); and 'should build on its reputation as leading the world in the appraisal of products to establish itself also as a world leader in promoting innovation and early adoption of treatments' (ibid.: 43).

While the issues under review by Cooksey and Kennedy were approached in a technocratic fashion, in the end they involve political choices as to what the NHS should provide in the way of treatments and interventions, and the resources required for such purposes. Such choices, and, more broadly, innovation as a fundamental value in NICE decision-making, are highly controversial, as Chapters 2, 5 and 6 make clear. In particular, working with the academic and pharmaceutical communities can give rise to conflicts of interest when those undertaking academic research have either held senior positions in pharmaceutical companies and/or receive funding for research, consultancies and speaking at conferences.

NICE has a clear conflicts of interest policy whereby those advising it are required to declare interests in an open and transparent manner. However, in practice achieving transparency and keeping the boundaries clear, especially in a highly charged political context, can be a challenge (and, on occasion, has led to litigation, as discussed in Chapter 9). A recent example concerns the arrival of a new weight-loss treatment to tackle obesity, known as Wegovy, which takes the form of an appetite-suppressing injection (Das and Ungoed-Thomas, 2023a and b). The leading obesity expert advocating the treatment and calling it a 'gamechanger' in the media turned out to have financial links to the Dutch company, Novo Nordisk, which developed the treatment. Others with financial links to the company gave evidence used by NICE in its decision to recommend the drug for use on the NHS. But it was claimed that 'despite potential conflicts of interest, the financial links were not always clear' (ibid.). NICE stated that it would assess whether its policies had been followed on this occasion.

The issue has particular political significance in a context where obesity rates in the UK are among the highest globally. The government has been under pressure for some time to tackle the issue by shifting the focus from individual behaviour and lifestyle changes to confronting the commercial determinants of health as part of a focus on improving population health. However, and in contrast to the devolved governments, there has been reluctance so far to introduce such policies in England on the grounds that they smack of the 'nanny state' and should be resisted. This is despite all the evidence that such policies work, in contrast to those focusing on individual behaviour which have limited impact at best. For a drug to appear at such a time and seemingly offering a quick fix to reduce weight therefore has a strong appeal to government (McCartney, 2023).

The Wegovy case illustrates a wider problem facing NICE and others engaged in getting evidence into policy and practice. Where the issue, as in the case of obesity and much else in public health, is a highly charged one politically, the role and impact of evidence on policy may prove limited, as discussed in Chapter 7. Reflecting on his time as a civil servant in the Cabinet Office, former academic Phil Davies points out the importance of the policy context, and indeed the political context, to understanding when and how evidence can be used (Davies, 2005). He goes on to argue (ibid.: 4) that:

> if you ask policy-makers where they go for their evidence, they will tell you that they go first to their special advisors, then to people who are called experts (in whom I have little faith), then to think-tanks and opinion formers, lobbyists and professional associations, media, their constituents, consumers and various users of services and only then, if they bother, will they turn to academics and research evidence. This point was also made by an internal piece of research in the Department of Trade and Industry in which a survey of their decision-makers found that academic research was not even mentioned.

While a great deal of academic literature has been produced since 2005 on getting evidence into policy and practice and how this can be improved or strengthened, it seems likely that Davies's description of how policy is informed (or not) by evidence remains valid.

Adopting a rather more instrumental approach to the challenge facing those seeking to get evidence into policy, the Chief Medical Officer for England, Chris Whitty, suggests that a key problem lies with the academic community which 'is often weak in producing papers usable in policy even when the evidence is there' (Whitty, 2015). In his view, academics fail to acknowledge the speed of the policy process and the need for papers which synthesise evidence from across different disciplines with an emphasis on economic analyses. However, if Davies's arguments remain valid, the challenge goes beyond how academic papers are crafted for policy purposes and entails the need for cultural change among officials and others seeking solutions to complex problems.

In this regard, the view advanced by Rutter and colleagues merits closer attention: if their analysis is correct then this is the context, often messy, with which NICE has to engage (Rutter et al., 2017). Tools and methods designed to answer questions about the effectiveness of clinical interventions are 'grounded in linear models of cause and effect' (ibid.). Public health problems by definition are complex and not solvable with a simple, single intervention. As the authors argue, much research funding and activity 'is heavily skewed towards studies that attempt to identify simple, often short-term, individual-level health outcomes, rather than complex, multiple, upstream, population-level actions and outcomes' (ibid.). This bias echoes the prioritisation favoured by policy-makers of individual-level interventions over system-level responses. Under such circumstances, and under successive governments of different political persuasions, 'lifestyle drift' triumphs over upstream interventions (Hunter et al., 2009). Redressing the imbalance demands 'reshaping public health research, policy and practice to incorporate complex systems approaches' (Rutter et al., 2017). But as NICE's experience in the public health domain, described in Chapter 7, clearly illustrates, this will always be a difficult task.

Another area where change affecting NICE is likely concerns the ongoing tension between national and local control. Like much of UK public policy-making, the emphasis in health policy is on top-down, command and control thinking with limited scope for local discretion or giving priority to local needs. Within the NHS, this battle has raged for much of its existence and remains alive. Most recently, the government commissioned a review of the new Integrated Care Systems (ICSs) being set up in England. It was led by a former Secretary of State for Health under New Labour, Patricia Hewitt. Its terms of reference focused on how much freedom locally is compatible with accountability; on how much space and time can be given to local leaders to lead; and on how a limited number of shared priorities can best be agreed. The report appeared in April 2023, and among its recommendations was a call for NHS England to be less punitive in holding ICSs to account, and less controlling by moving away from the traditional top-down approach to which the NHS has become accustomed (Hewitt, 2023). Hewitt favoured a bottom-up approach where local areas, paying attention to their particular contexts, find solutions to local problems. The centre's role becomes one of facilitating change – providing implementation support, training and learning to assist local organisations in meeting their goals.

NICE operates in a world where for much of its work, a national focus is paramount. If there is to be a move to greater local autonomy and variation, this will have implications for NICE's operating model and how it interacts with local systems. To a degree, its work in public health and social care requires working with local government where there is much variation. Perhaps there are lessons from this part of its portfolio which might be applied more widely.

Conclusion

We have argued here that NICE has survived in large part by being a responsive, listening organisation. It has heeded concerns of critics and commentators (several of whom have contributed to this book), has sought to involve stakeholders in its work, and evolved its methods accordingly over the quarter-century of its existence to date.

However, a key risk for any organisation which adapts in this manner is: at what stage does it cease to be the organisation it was at the beginning? The danger is that, in the process of evolution, NICE may lose the identity, status and legitimacy that it has possessed for most of its lifetime to date, both in the UK and globally. Some already argue that point is close to being reached (Michaels, 2023).

Yet, whether NICE remains the same organisation in structural and process terms into the future is less significant than ensuring that its culture – one of responsiveness, inclusivity and a solid grounding in evidence – remains intact and is not eroded. Structures and processes are bound to change to meet new objectives and changing circumstances, including those identified in this book. This is no bad thing, because it helps an organisation to avoid becoming static, complacent or irrelevant. But if the key cultural features which have ensured both NICE's survival and success can be retained and protected, there is no reason to presume that it cannot endure, and prosper, for another 25 years.

References

BBC News (2013) 'Stafford Hospital: "I am truly sorry" – David Cameron' (6 February). Available at: https://www.bbc.co.uk/news/av/uk-politics-21348901 (Accessed 16 April 2023).

Blair, T. and Hague, W. (2023) *A New National Purpose: Innovation Can Power the Future of Britain*. London: Tony Blair Institute for Global Change.

Cooksey, D. (2006) *A Review of UK Health Research Funding*. London: HMSO.

Das, S, and Ungoed-Thomas, J. (2023a) 'Revealed: experts who praised new "skinny jab" funded by drug maker', *The Observer* (12 March). Available at: https://www.theguardian.com/business/2023/mar/12/revealed-experts-who-praised-new-skinny-jab-received-payments-from-drug-maker#:~:text=The%20Observer%20can%20reveal%3A3,3.6m%20by%20the%20firm (Accessed 15 April 2023).

Das S and Ungoed-Thomas J (2023b) '"Skinny jab" drug firm facing fresh inquiries after "serious breaches" of industry code', *The Observer* (19 March). Available at: https://www.theguardian.com/business/2023/mar/18/skinny-jab-drug-firm-facing-fresh-inquiries-after-breach-of-industry-code#:~:text=The%20action%20on%20Thursday%20followed,weight%2Dloss%20drugs%2C%20Saxenda (Accessed 15 April 2023).

Davies, P. (2005) 'Evidence-based policy at the Cabinet Office'. Impact and Insight Seminar, Overseas Development Institute (17 October). Available at: https://slideplayer.com/slide/6292/ (Accessed 12 April 2023).

Francis, R. (2012) *Report of the Mid-Staffordshire NHS Foundation Trust Public Inquiry*. Available at: https://www.gov.uk/government/publications/report-of-the-mid-stafford shire-nhs-foundation-trust-public-inquiry (Accessed 23 October 2023).

Hewitt, P. (2023) *The Hewitt Review. An Independent Review of Integrated Care Systems*. Available at: https://assets.publishing.service.gov.uk/media/642b07d87de82b00123134fa/the-hewitt-review.pdf (Accessed 15 April 2023).

Hunter, D.J., Popay, J., Tannahill, C., Whitehead, M. and Elson, T. (2009) *Learning the Lessons from the Past: Shaping a Different Future*. Available at: http://www.institute-ofhealthequity.org/resources-reports/the-marmot-review-working-committee-3-report (Accessed 18 April 2023).

Kennedy, I. (2009) *Appraising the Value of Innovation and other Benefits. A Short Study for NICE*. London: NICE.

Klein, R. and Maybin, J. (2012) *Thinking about Rationing*. London: The King's Fund.

Labour Party (2023) *5 Missions for a Better Britain*. London: Labour Party.

Littlejohns, P., Weale, A., Chalkidou, K., Faden, R. and Teerwattananon, Y. (2012) 'Social values and health policy: a new international research programme', *Journal of Health Organization and Management*, 26(3), pp.285–92.

Littlejohns P., Knight, A., Littlejohns, A., Poole, T-L. and Kieslich, K. (2017) 'Setting standards and monitoring quality in the NHS 1999–2013: a classic case of goal conflict', *International Journal of Health Planning and Management*, 32(2), pp.e185–e205.

Littlejohns, P., Kieslich, K., Weale, A., Tumilty, E., Richrdson, G., Stokes, T., Gauld, R. and Scuffham, P. (2019a) 'Creating sustainable health care systems: Agreeing social (societal) priorities through public participation', *Journal of Health Organization and Management*, 33(1), pp.18–34.

Littlejohns, P., Chalkidou, K., Culyer, A.J., Weale, A., Rid, A., Kieslich, K., Coultas, C., Max, C. et al. (2019b) 'National Institute for Health and Care Excellence, social values and healthcare priority setting', *Journal of the Royal Society of Medicine*, 112(5), pp.113–19.

Littlejohns, P., Hunter, D.J., Weale, A., Johnson, J. and Khatun, T. (2024) *Making Health Public: A Manifesto for a New Social Contract*. Bristol: Policy Press.

McCartney, M. (2023) 'Medicine and the media: semaglutide: should the media slim down its enthusiasm?', *British Medical Journal*, 380, p.624.

Michaels, A.J. (2023) 'Is NICE losing its standing as a trusted source of guidance?', *British Medical Journal*, 383, p.2751

NICE (2008) *Social Value Judgements*. 2nd edn. London: NICE.

NICE (2020) *Our Principles: The Principles that Guide the Development of NICE Guidance and Standards*. London: NICE.

Rutter, H., Savona, N., Glonti, K., Bibby, J., Cummins, S. and Finegood, D.T. (2017) 'The need for a complex systems model of evidence for public health', *The Lancet*, 390(10112), pp.2602–04.

Smith, R. (2000) 'The failings of NICE: time to start work on version 2', *British Medical Journal*, 321(7273), pp.1363–64.

Smith, R. (2004) 'The triumph of NICE', *British Medical Journal*, 329(7459).

Sylvester, R. (2023) 'What is the *Times* Health Commission? Its aims explained', *The Times* (15 January). Available at: https://www.thetimes.co.uk/article/times-health-commission-explained-objective-commissioners-bvl2937gf (Accessed 20 April 2023).

Syrett, K. (2003) 'A technocratic fix to the 'legitimacy problem'? The Blair Government and Healthcare Rationing in the United Kingdom', *Journal of Health Politics, Policy and Law*, 28(4), pp.715–46.

Weale, A., Kieslich, K., Littlejohns, P., Tugendhaft, A., Tumilty, E., Weerasuriya, K. and Whitty, J.A. (2016) 'Priority setting, equitable access and public involvement in health care', *Journal of Health Organization and Management*, 30(5), pp.736–50.

Whitty, C.J.M. (2015) 'What makes an academic paper useful for health policy?', *BMC Medicine* 13, p.301.

Index

For Product Safety Concerns and Information please contact our EU
representative GPSR@taylorandfrancis.com
Taylor & Francis Verlag GmbH, Kaufingerstraße 24, 80331 München, Germany